PHARMACOLOGY - RESEARCH, SAFETY TESTING AND REGULATION

BUPRENORPHINE

PHARMACOLOGY, CLINICAL USES AND POTENTIAL SIDE EFFECTS

PHARMACOLOGY - RESEARCH, SAFETY TESTING AND REGULATION

Additional books in this series can be found on Nova's website under the Series tab.

Additional e-books in this series can be found on Nova's website under the e-book tab.

PHARMACOLOGY - RESEARCH, SAFETY TESTING AND REGULATION

BUPRENORPHINE

PHARMACOLOGY, CLINICAL USES AND POTENTIAL SIDE EFFECTS

ROSALINA BENNET
EDITOR

nova publishers
New York

For permission to use material from this book please contact us:
Telephone 631-231-7269; Fax 631-231-8175
Web Site: http://www.novapublishers.com

Additional color graphics may be available in the e-book version of this book.

Library of Congress Cataloging-in-Publication Data

ISBN: 978-1-63321-136-0

Library of Congress Control Number: 2014940579

Published by Nova Science Publishers, Inc. † New York

CONTENTS

PREFACE

This book begins by reviewing the pharmacology of buprenorphine and co-ingredient naloxone; its use in addiction medicine and pain management; and clinical challenges, with special emphasis on drug-drug interactions (pharmacokinetic and pharmacodynamic), safety concerns, and buprenorphine misuse. The book continues to discuss the role of buprenorphine as an analgesic; the application of buprenorphone in acute and chronic pancreatitis; and the substitution maintenance treatment of opioid dependence with buprenorphine and naloxone.

Chapter 1 – Buprenorphine was introduced in the United States as an injectable analgesic in 1981 and treatment option for opioid dependence in 2002; a transdermal formulation was approved for pain management in 2010. Following the introduction of this variety of dosage forms, buprenorphine use and misuse have increased significantly. This article reviews the pharmacology of buprenorphine and co-ingredient naloxone; use in addiction medicine and pain management; and clinical challenges, with special emphasis on drug-drug interactions (pharmacokinetic and pharmacodynamic), safety concerns, and buprenorphine misuse. Buprenorphine accessibility for nonmedical use is widespread in some settings, and burgeoning prescription and abuse rates have led to multiple reports of overdoses and fatalities associated with its use. Buprenorphine abuse potential, prevalence and patterns of misuse, and risk factors associated with fatal overdose are discussed. Given the epidemic of prescription drug misuse, practitioners have an increasing need for clinical monitoring for compliance and misuse of controlled substances, including buprenorphine. Most guidelines recommend urine drug testing, but monitoring of buprenorphine presents special challenges to laboratories and practitioners interpreting results. Compliance and abuse monitoring for buprenorphine may be performed by different test methodologies, with immunoassay and mass spectrometry methods in most frequent use; each technology offers unique advantages and disadvantages. Testing of other specimen types for buprenorphine including blood, oral fluid, hair, sweat, breath, and meconium is feasible. The disposition of buprenorphine and its metabolites in each specimen type varies and may impact specific testing methodology. Interpreting drug tests requires understanding of buprenorphine's unique properties and factors that influence detection. Considerations include metabolic and dispositional patterns in tissues, and differences in the use of specific formulations or routes of administration (e.g., injection, sublingual, or transdermal) for specific applications.

Chapter 2 – Potent opioids have different efficacy, particularly opioids such as buprenorphine may have advantages due to unique pharmacodynamics and pharmacokinetics. Prospective studies have demonstrated the benefits to buprenorphine in several clinical situations. However, randomized control trials are few and far between and need to be done to demonstrate these advantages. Buprenorphine appears to be a safe potent opioid with few drug interactions and reduced risk for respiratory, cardiac, gastrointestinal, sexual and cognitive adverse effects. Certain populations and clinical situations favor the use of buprenorphine as a first line opioid.

Chapter 3 – Buprenorphine is a semi-synthetic derivate of thebaine. Buprenorphine has both analgesic and antihyperalgesic systemic effects but the exact mechanism of the different modalities remains unknown. It has three known receptor binding mechanisms. First Buprenorphine is an μ-opioid receptor agonist. Secondly Buprenorphine shows partial agonistic activity at the opioid receptor-like receptor 1 (ORL1)-receptor that induces a pronociceptive effect, for example useful in the treatment of hyperalgesia. Its antagonistic activity at the third receptor, the κ-opioid receptor, might explain the less sedative and psychomimetic effects compared to morphine or fentanyl.

Buprenorphine is metabolised by the liver into norbuprenorphine. The latter is a μ-opioid, δ-opioid and nociception receptor full agonist, as well as a κ-opioid receptor partial agonist. After glucuronidation, both glucuronides are eliminated mainly through excretion into the bile.

A higher-dose sublingual form (up to 2 mg) is indicated for detoxification and long-term replacement therapy in opioid dependency. It is also a good alternative to sustained–release opioids such as morphine and oxycodone. The transdermal form is indicated for the treatment of severe cancer pain and severe non-cancer pain not responding to non-opioids. But also in orthopaedic surgery e.g., in elderly, it is proven an effective tool for pain control. The intravenous formulation is used in continuous postoperative pain treatment.

Conflicting results have been published on the efficacy and duration of various opioids (including buprenorphine) in prolonging the duration of local anaesthetics. The regional use of buprenorphine has been described in neuraxial and peripheral blocks as adjuvants. Local buprenorphine application, e.g., to the stellate ganglion, is also described in chronical pain management.

Buprenorphine can be sleep-inducing which can be an advantage when pain is accompanied with sleeplessness. Other clinical indications are pregnancy, maxillofacial surgery, treatment in non-suicidal self-injury, vasectomy surgery, and due the euphoria and anxiolytic effects it can be used as an alternative antidepressant in patients with depression due to pain.

The adverse effects are similar to those of other opioids. The most important side effect is nausea and vomiting, in particular when initiated at high doses.

Another important side- effect is respiratory depression but due to a relatively long half-life, this depression is characterised by a ceiling effect. The combination with alcohol and/or benzodiazepines however, can lead to fatal respiratory depression.

A "precipitated withdrawal" is described when buprenorphine is used in persons with a physically dependency for full-agonist opioids, who are not already in withdrawal.

Buprenorphine is a common used opioid that provide effective pain relief in cancer and non-cancer patients. As an adjuvant used in regional anesthesia, it is likely to? prolong the peripheral nerve block duration.

Chapter 4 – Pancreatitis is an inflammation of the pancreas. The most common causes are alcohol consumption and gallstone related. Interestingly, pancreatitis is the most incidence observed in patients following abdominal surgery. The most frequently symptoms of pancreatitis are severe abdominal pain, nausea and vomiting. Heart and respiratory function may also be affected. How to reasonably choose a safe, effective and low-dependent analgesic is a big problem faced by the doctors. Analgesics will not affect the recovery of the disease if the patients have chronic or acute inflammation, however it will release the symptoms and make the patients more comfortable. In general, more than one type of analgesics are used in treating pancreatitis, such as acetaminophen, non-steroidal anti-inflammatory drug and opioid etc., which is greatly controversial in clinical application because of the side effects such as ulcers associated with their use. In addition, some studies have shown that the use of opioid may conceal the changes of the disease and because their spasmogenic effects will increase the patients' ache, this in turn increases the sphincter pressure of oddi in abdominal cavity. The biliary tract pressure increase seems to be related with dosage and plasma concentration of opioid and seems to be apparently regulated by the Mu (μ) receptor.

There is a subclass of opioid drug called buprenorphine hydrochloride, along with its relatively outstanding pharmacologic character to be gradually known. buprenorphine can be used as substitute for the drug dolantin in treating the abdominal ache associated with acute and chronic pancreatitis. The use of burprenorphine can be an alternative choice to treat the aching of acute pancreatitis which has less side effects. Compared with other analgesia plans, buprenorphine can reduce analgesia metering needed, and which has no obvious differences in the risk of both the appearances of pancreatitis complication and clinical adverse events. According to the current clinical studies, buprenorphine is the suitable choice for treating the aching of acute pancreatitis, and compared with other analgesia drugs that are not belonging to opioid category. Currently for acute paroxysm associated with chronic pancreatitis, the common suggestions for treatment do not provide enough analgesia effect. Therefore the German Guide suggest the use of dolantin, buprenorphine and procaine administered intravenously as a treatment plan for the abdominal pain resulting from pancreatitis. It is very difficult to control the intractable aching of chronic pancreatitis, but fortunately, it has been reported that buprenorphine is very effective in alleviating the pain that is felt by the patients with chronic pancreatitis. The use of buprenorphine is a simple, safe and effective way compared with current drugs used in treating abdominal ache as a result of pancreatitis.

Chapter 5 – *Aim:* To present medical assisted treatment of opiate dependence with substitution medicament Buprenorphine/Naloxone (Suboxone®) in Bosnia and Herzegovina, with which we may prevent social excluding of young individuals who were opiate dependants.

General overview: Until recently there was no solution for long-term and comprehensive treatment of young persons who suffer from opiate dependency. This is not illness that impairs only psychical health of addicts with possible life threatening consequences, but this is serious problem in whole society because of aftereffects that lead young people in social excluding: delinquencies, criminals, violations and imprisonments. In health care institutions there are no capacities for the stationary treatment for longer term, what is necessary for the treatment of drug dependence, and less adequate solution is seating in penal and upbringing institutions, which, besides stigmatizing young protégés, it excludes young addicts from normal social life in addition. The most modern medically assisted method of substitution treatment of opiate dependants with medical substance Buprenorphine/Naloxone (Suboxone®) has been implemented. This medicament with its characteristics offers possibility for out-patient treatment. With this it is possible to achieve prompt and effective results of detoxification and weaning of opiates. Treated opiate dependants become “clear minded”, qualified for the all professional and social activities, what improves significantly quality of family and social relationship. With this way the treatment in the institutions can be avoided, therefore it preventing social excluding of young person’s treated with this method.

Conclusion: Medical assisted treatment of opiate dependence with Buprenorphine/Naloxone is implementing outpatient program with involvement of close family members who are not drug dependants. It brings back “clear mind” to treated young opiate addicts, it does not stigmatize but it re-socialize and in that way it is preventing social excluding of young opiate dependant persons.

In: Buprenorphine
Editor: Rosalina Bennet
ISBN: 978-1-63321-136-0

Chapter 1

BUPRENORPHINE: CLINICAL USE, ABUSE AND COMPLIANCE MONITORING

Anne Z. DePriest, Pharm.D., BCPS[1,*], Katie Miller, Pharm.D., BCPS[1] and Edward J. Cone, Ph.D.[2]

[1]Aegis Sciences Corporation, Nashville, Tennessee; The University of Tennessee Health Science Center, College of Pharmacy, Memphis, Tennessee, US

[2]Johns Hopkins School of Medicine, Department of Psychiatry and Behavioral Sciences, Baltimore, Maryland, US

ABSTRACT

Buprenorphine was introduced in the United States as an injectable analgesic in 1981 and treatment option for opioid dependence in 2002; a transdermal formulation was approved for pain management in 2010. Following the introduction of this variety of dosage forms, buprenorphine use and misuse have increased significantly. This article reviews the pharmacology of buprenorphine and co-ingredient naloxone; use in addiction medicine and pain management; and clinical challenges, with special emphasis on drug-drug interactions (pharmacokinetic and pharmacodynamic), safety concerns, and buprenorphine misuse. Buprenorphine accessibility for nonmedical use is widespread in some settings, and burgeoning prescription and abuse rates have led to multiple reports of overdoses and fatalities associated with its use. Buprenorphine

* E-mail: anne.depriest@aegislabs.com, annedepriest@gmail.com.

abuse potential, prevalence and patterns of misuse, and risk factors associated with fatal overdose are discussed. Given the epidemic of prescription drug misuse, practitioners have an increasing need for clinical monitoring for compliance and misuse of controlled substances, including buprenorphine. Most guidelines recommend urine drug testing, but monitoring of buprenorphine presents special challenges to laboratories and practitioners interpreting results. Compliance and abuse monitoring for buprenorphine may be performed by different test methodologies, with immunoassay and mass spectrometry methods in most frequent use; each technology offers unique advantages and disadvantages. Testing of other specimen types for buprenorphine including blood, oral fluid, hair, sweat, breath, and meconium is feasible. The disposition of buprenorphine and its metabolites in each specimen type varies and may impact specific testing methodology. Interpreting drug tests requires understanding of buprenorphine's unique properties and factors that influence detection. Considerations include metabolic and dispositional patterns in tissues, and differences in the use of specific formulations or routes of administration (e.g., injection, sublingual, or transdermal) for specific applications.

INTRODUCTION

Buprenorphine is an opioid analgesic prepared from thebaine, and is similar in structure to other phenanthrene-derivative opiates including codeine and morphine [1]. First synthesized in 1966, it has been available since the 1970s as an analgesic [2-4]. A parenteral dosage form was approved in the U.S. in 1981 and first marketed in 1985 as a Schedule V drug under the Controlled Substances Act [2-3, 5]. In 2002, buprenorphine sublingual (SL) tablets were approved in the U.S. for the treatment of opioid dependence, and reclassified as Schedule III controlled substances [5-6]. Other formulations in the U.S. have been subsequently introduced, and today buprenorphine is available in more than 40 countries [7].

Buprenorphine is used extensively worldwide for the treatment of opioid dependence and pain management, with increasing use in the U.S. in recent years. Its unique pharmacologic and pharmacokinetic profile creates effects that vary significantly from other opioids, which may be advantageous or disadvantageous depending on the circumstance. Buprenorphine is also subject to abuse, as evidenced by numerous reports of diversion and fatal overdose. This chapter reviews the clinical uses of buprenorphine, safety considerations, abuse potential, and methods of toxicological analysis.

PHARMACOLOGY

Buprenorphine exerts opioid activity as a partial agonist at mu opioid receptors and antagonist at kappa opioid receptors [6]. Mu receptor agonism mediates supraspinal analgesia, respiratory depression, and miosis, while kappa receptor antagonism results in limited spinal analgesia, dysphoria, and psychomimetic effects [2]. Buprenorphine has a high affinity for delta opioid receptors where it is thought to act as an agonist, though its effect is poorly understood [2, 8]. Some investigators have suggested buprenorphine is actually a delta receptor antagonist, and central nervous system (CNS) delta receptor upregulation has been demonstrated following buprenorphine administration in animal models [9-10]. Both delta agonist and antagonist effects have been observed *in vivo*, with agonist effects apparent only under some conditions and with lower potency than mu- or kappa-mediated effects [10]. Partial agonist activity has also been demonstrated at the ORL-1 (nociceptin) receptor, which may contribute to analgesia by a non-opioid mechanism [8, 11]. The rewarding effects of buprenorphine are mediated by mu and delta receptor agonism and kappa receptor antagonism [12]. It has also been theorized that norbuprenorphine, a metabolite of buprenorphine, may exert higher activity at delta receptors than the parent compound [10].

The dose response curve for buprenorphine has been described as biphasic or even triphasic [11]. In animal studies, peak effects were demonstrated at subcutaneous (SC) doses between 0.25 and 0.5 mg/kg (agonist phase), with decreasing effects noted up to 10 mg/kg (antagonist phase). A second increase in analgesia was observed in higher doses [13-17]. Noncompetitive inhibition is theorized to contribute to the bell-shaped dose response curve observed with buprenorphine. At low doses, agonism at one receptor site increases analgesia; at high doses, interaction with a second receptor of lower affinity counteracts the effects of the first [16]. It is possible the antagonist phase observed with buprenorphine doses greater than 0.5 mg/kg is related to ORL-1 agonism [18].

The pharmacologic activity of buprenorphine is variably more potent than morphine, depending on dose and effect; buprenorphine was demonstrated to be 10 times more potent than morphine in a formalin test, and 25 to 50 times more potent as an analgesic on a per mg basis [1-2, 19]. An analgesic effect may be observed with 5% to 10% mu receptor occupancy [14]. Continual increases in mu receptor binding are demonstrable up to doses of 32 mg SL, at which point receptor occupancy is near maximum [20]. Buprenorphine has a very high affinity and slow dissociation from mu receptors, leading to a long duration of action [21-22]. Buprenorphine mediated analgesia is not related to plasma concentrations, because dissociation from CNS opioid receptors lags behind clearance from the plasma compartment [23]. Consequently, subjective and physiologic effects can persist up to three days following sublingual administration [24]. The antagonist potency of buprenorphine is thought to be equivalent to naltrexone [1].

Naloxone is a competitive opioid antagonist, and is added to some sublingual formulations of buprenorphine [4]. It does not exert any intrinsic activity [2].

Pharmacokinetics

Absorption

Buprenorphine has limited bioavailability by the oral route due to high first-pass metabolism, with only 15% of a dose reaching systemic circulation [25]. Due to high lipid solubility, buprenorphine may be administered sublingually, bypassing first-pass metabolism and resulting in 28% to 55% bioavailability [2, 25-28].

The portion of a dose that is swallowed is only minimally absorbed, which contributes to significant variability in absorption following sublingual administration [29]. Sublingual bioavailability is also influenced by pH; because buprenorphine is a weak base, more drug is non-ionized at high pH and absorption is enhanced [30-31].

Sublingual absorption is rapid, and buprenorphine is deposited into oral mucosa within 5 minutes [30]. Absorption from the mucosa into systemic circulation occurs much more slowly [31]. An initial study demonstrated a mean time to peak plasma concentrations of 200 minutes, with a range of 1.5 to 6 hours [25]. The analytical technique used to measure plasma concentrations was achieved by radioimmunoassay, which cannot distinguish between buprenorphine and norbuprenorphine. With improved analysis by mass spectrometry techniques, peak plasma concentrations could be more accurately measured in later studies. Apparent peak plasma concentrations occur earlier than previously published, though still with significant variability (40 minutes to 3.5 hours) [31-34]. Less variability is noted with chronic dosing, potentially due to the existence of buprenorphine as a drug reservoir in oral mucosa, with peak concentrations occurring between 1 and 2 hours [31, 35]. Peak effects after sublingual administration occur between 3 and 7 hours [36].

Parenteral administration may result in variable absorption by the intramuscular (IM) route, with bioavailability reported between 40% to 90% [2]. Peak effects following intravenous (IV) administration occur between 15 minutes and 3 hours [36]. Transdermal absorption of buprenorphine yields 15% bioavailability for all doses. Buprenorphine permeates intact skin, producing detectable plasma concentrations at a 25 pg/mL threshold with a median time of 17 hours [8].

Steady-state plasma concentrations in the pg/mL range are reached within 48 hours, with a time to maximum concentrations of approximately 72 hours [37]. Intranasal administration results in rapid absorption and avoidance of first-pass metabolism, resulting in 38% to 50% bioavailability similar to sublingual dosing. Maximal plasma concentrations are reached with 10 to 40 minutes [2, 38-39].

Naloxone has negligible bioavailability when administered orally or sublingually [6]. Intranasal absorption is enhanced, with 24% to 30% bioavailability following administration of 0.5 mg or 2 mg doses [39]. Its addition to sublingual buprenorphine formulations is intended to provide an abuse-deterrent effect, as it may exert opioid antagonism and precipitate withdrawal following parenteral or intranasal administration [6, 28, 40-42].

Distribution

Buprenorphine may extensively distribute to adipose tissue due to its high lipophilicity, yielding a large volume of distribution of approximately 430 L [2].

It is 96% bound to plasma proteins including alpha- and beta-globulin [6, 8]. Distribution to the brain occurs rapidly following intravenous use, with a brain-to-plasma ratio of 3 observed as quickly as 15 minutes post-administration and up to 10.5 at 6 hours in animal studies [43-44]. Conversely, buprenorphine concentrations in cerebrospinal fluid are 15% to 25% of concurrent plasma concentrations following transdermal administration [8]. Norbuprenorphine exerts low permeability across the blood-brain-barrier, with brain-to-plasma ratios less than 0.1 [31, 45]. However, norbuprenorphine has been detected in postmortem cases following overdose, indicating potential involvement and saturation of a transporter system such as P-glycoprotein [31]. Naloxone is approximately 45% protein bound, primarily to albumin, and results in low plasma concentrations following sublingual administration [6, 31, 46].

Metabolism

Buprenorphine undergoes extensive Phase I and II metabolism by cytochrome P450 (CYP450) and UDP-glucuronosyltransferase (UGT) enzymes, respectively [47]. Buprenorphine is N-dealkylated primarily by CYP3A4 to norbuprenorphine, with some involvement from CYP2C8 [27, 48-49]. *In vitro* data suggests that 65% of norbuprenorphine formation is due to CYP3A4, with CYP2C8 accounting for 30%. Minor roles for other CYP2C enzymes including CYP2C9, 2C19, and 2C18 have also been demonstrated, with no activity of CYP2D6 and CYP2E1 reported [50]. Both buprenorphine and norbuprenorphine undergo glucuronidation, with conjugation of buprenorphine to buprenorphine-3-beta-O-glucuronide primarily by UGT2B7 with a lesser role for UGT1A1, and conjugation of norbuprenorphine by UGT1A3 and less by UGT1A1 [51-52]. Metabolism of buprenorphine is 100-fold greater in the liver than small intestine. Phase II glucuronidation may occur in both the liver and small intestine, with no observed differences in rates [45]. The metabolites of buprenorphine are largely active. Norbuprenorphine possesses 25% of the intrinsic activity of buprenorphine. However, due to its limited transport across the blood-brain-barrier, its contribution to analgesic efficacy is limited to approximately 2% [44]. The glucuronide conjugates bind to opioid receptors, with possible contribution to antinociception, decreased tidal volume, and sedation [53]. Up to five hydroxylated metabolites have been more recently identified, with metabolites M1 and M2 as hydroxylated forms of buprenorphine and M3, M4, and M5 as hydroxylated norbuprenorphine. Buprenorphine is first metabolized to M1 and M2, which may undergo subsequent N-dealkylation to the other metabolites. Metabolism of norbuprenorphine may also lead directly to M3 formation [51]. The formation of M1 appears to be mediated by CYP3A4 and CYP2C8, and M3 from buprenorphine and norbuprenorphine via CYP3A4/5 [49, 51]. Both metabolites undergo glucuronidation, with more extensive metabolism of M1 than M3 [49]. M1 and M3 have been detected in human urine, primarily in conjugated forms [51]. Buprenorphine metabolism pathways are illustrated in Figure 1.

Metabolism of buprenorphine from transdermal administration is negligible in skin [8]. Sex-related differences in metabolism have been described, with higher plasma area under the curve (AUC) values and maximum concentrations for buprenorphine, norbuprenorphine, and norbuprenorphine-glucuronide in females. AUC relative to dose per body weight and surface area was higher for norbuprenorphine.

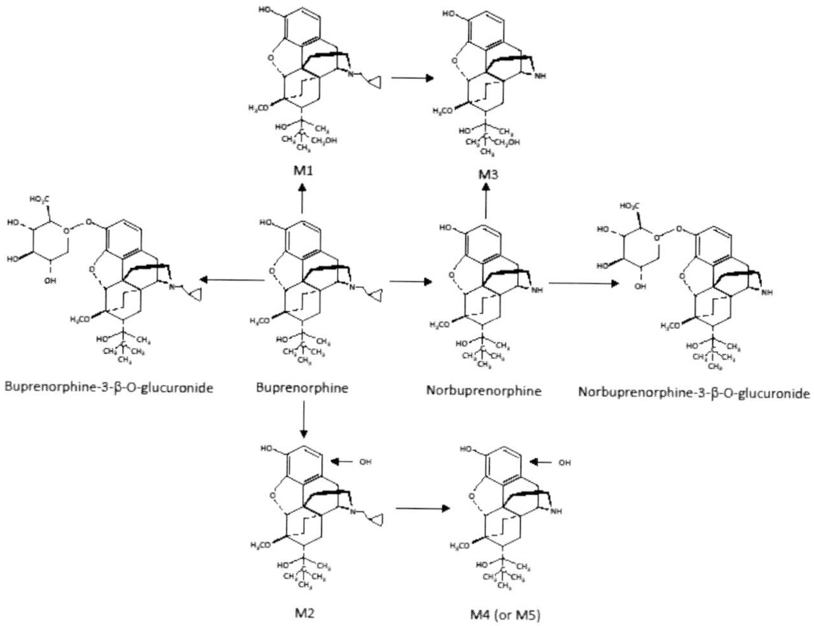

Figure 1. Metabolism of buprenorphine [1, 49, 51].

It is possible that differences in body composition and CYP3A-dependent metabolism may contribute to these findings [54].

Naloxone undergoes N-dealkylation via CYP2C18 and CYP2C19, with lower contribution from CYP3A4 and CYP2D6, to nornaloxone; nornaloxone is also known as noroxymorphone, the metabolite of oxymorphone and noroxycodone (a metabolite of oxycodone) [55-56]. Naloxone is additionally metabolized by reduction of the 6-oxo group to naloxol, and undergoes glucuronidation along with two metabolites [35, 57].

Excretion

Buprenorphine is excreted by biliary and renal routes, with 70% of the dose in feces and 27% to 30% in urine [6, 45, 47, 58]. Urinary elimination occurs for up to 11 days, with 1% as free buprenorphine, 9.4% as buprenorphine-glucuronide, 2.7% as free norbuprenorphine, and 11% as norbuprenorphine-glucuronide [6, 47, 58]. Total clearance is 55 L/hour in postoperative patients [8]. Buprenorphine follows a three compartment pharmacokinetic model, with biphasic or triphasic elimination [2, 45, 59]. Enterohepatic circulation is evidenced by increased concentrations of buprenorphine and metabolites appearing 4 to 6 days post-dose when urine concentrations of conjugated buprenorphine are low [47, 58].

Due to the complexity of elimination, reported half-lives of buprenorphine and norbuprenorphine are highly variable in literature and influenced by both assay sensitivity and route of administration. Sublingual administration resulting in drug depot and sequestration in adipose tissue can result in longer elimination half-lives than those observed following parenteral administration [31]. Very short half-lives after intravenous use were reported, with an initial half-life of 2 minutes and a mean terminal half-life of 5 hours; another study cited a terminal half-life of 3.2 hours, and a range of 1.6 to 8.2 hours [25-26]. Elimination half-lives following sublingual administration have been reported between 3 and 44 hours [31]. Regardless, the half-lives of both buprenorphine and norbuprenorphine typically exceed 24 hours, with 37 hours for the sublingual tablet and 24 to 48 hours for the sublingual film cited in manufacturer prescribing information [6, 24, 31, 45]. Following removal of the transdermal patch, mean buprenorphine plasma concentrations decrease by half within 10 to 24 hours, with a terminal half-life of 26 hours [8]. Norbuprenorphine has a longer terminal half-life than buprenorphine and may accumulate with chronic dosing [26].

Naloxone has a much shorter elimination half-life than buprenorphine, ranging from 1 to 2 hours intravenously and 2 to 12 hours sublingually. Naloxone's lower plasma concentrations thus also decline more quickly than buprenorphine [6, 31, 35, 46]. The addition of naloxone to combination sublingual tablets does not affect the pharmacokinetics of buprenorphine [31].

AVAILABLE FORMULATIONS

Buprenorphine is currently available worldwide as parenteral, sublingual, and transdermal formulations. The parenteral formulation Buprenex® (Reckitt Benckiser, U.S.) contains buprenorphine 0.3 ng/mL and is administered in doses of 0.3 to 0.6 mg IV/IM for analgesia [60]. Buprenorphine is available in a variety of sublingual formulations. A sublingual tablet including buprenorphine alone was first marketed as Subutex® (Reckitt Benckiser, U.S.) 2 mg and 8 mg for the treatment of opioid dependence; the brand was discontinued in 2011 due to abuse concerns [61]. A combination tablet containing buprenorphine/naloxone was marketed initially as Suboxone® (Reckitt Benckiser, U.S.) in 2 mg/0.5 mg and 8 mg/2 mg strengths, also for the treatment of opioid dependence; it too was discontinued in 2013 following pediatric exposures resulting in fatal overdose [62]. The 4:1 ratio of buprenorphine to naloxone was selected to attenuate opioid effects without inducing withdrawal [63]. Generic formulations are still available for both the mono- and combination-products. Reformulated combination buprenorphine/ naloxone sublingual tablets marketed as Zubsolv® (Orexo, U.S.) in 1.4 mg/0.36 mg and 5.7 mg/1.4 mg strengths are currently available, though they are not equivalent in bioavailability to former preparations, and most closely equate to generic 2 mg/0.5 mg and 8 mg/2 mg dosage strengths, respectively. Naloxone exhibits a 12% lower bioavailability with this formulation [64]. Suboxone® (buprenorphine/naloxone) sublingual film (Reckitt Benckiser, U.S.) was approved in the U.S. in 2010 in dosages of 2 mg/0.5 mg, 4 mg/1 mg, 8 mg/2 mg, and 12 mg/3 mg [65]. The film dissolves more quickly than the tablets, and tamper-proof packaging reduces accidental exposure by children [66]. The transdermal buprenorphine patch was approved in the U.S. in 2010 as Butrans® (Purdue Pharma, U.S.) 5 mcg/hour, 10 mcg/hour, and 20 mcg/hour for once weekly administration [8]. This formulation is the first indicated for pain management since the introduction of parenteral buprenorphine thirty years ago, though the sublingual formulations have been used off-label for this purpose.

A buprenorphine subdermal implant has been investigated in the U.S. for the treatment of opioid dependence. Implantable buprenorphine was first studied in the 1980s in animal studies [67]. This unique formulation could yield benefits including decreased diversion and abuse, and prevention of accidental ingestion by children. The formulation Probuphine® (Titan Pharmaceutials, U.S.) is designed as a small, solid rod containing ethylene-vinyl acetate and buprenorphine in a solid matrix; two to four rods are administered in the upper inner arm in an office procedure, and removed at the end of a 6-month treatment period. Buprenorphine is designed to release slowly through dissolution, making it the first long-acting buprenorphine formulation [68]. The first double-blind, placebo-controlled study with buprenorphine subdermal implants was published in 2010. The implantation of four rods following induction with sublingual buprenorphine was associated with less use of illicit drugs compared to placebo, with a significantly lower incidence of illicit positive urine toxicology results during weeks 1 through 16. Retention was better for the buprenorphine implant group versus placebo, but 34% withdrew from the buprenorphine group [69]. The new drug application

(NDA) was submitted to the U.S. Food and Drug Administration (FDA) in October 2012 and given priority review; however, the NDA was rejected in April 2013. The FDA has requested additional data, specifically regarding the ability of the formulation to provide opioid blockade of relevant doses of mu agonists; the effect of higher doses to more closely approximate plasma levels associated with buprenorphine 12-16 mg/day SL; and human factors testing of training for insertion and removal of the implant [70].

When injected, naloxone may attenuate the euphoric effects of buprenorphine, which may in turn reduce the abuse liability of combination products [71]. Its deterrent value has been questioned, as buprenorphine has a considerably higher affinity for mu receptors than naloxone, and is not easily displaced [22]. In nondependent heroin abusers, reinforcing effects did not differ between buprenorphine/naloxone and buprenorphine alone [72]. Nevertheless, multiple studies demonstrate that naloxone precipitates withdrawal in opioid dependent subjects if injected with buprenorphine/ naloxone sublingual tablets [73-76]. Some investigators have theorized that low amounts of sublingual absorption of naloxone may have a minor impact on patients switching from buprenorphine monotherapy to a combination product. In one study, half of subjects experienced adverse reactions following transition; this was a retrospective study and subjects were not blinded, thus failing to rule out subjective effects of the participants [77]. No difference in treatment outcomes has been demonstrated between the buprenorphine mono-product and the combination sublingual tablets with naloxone [78]. Patients may prefer the combination product for palatability and disintegration time [79].

Some buprenorphine formulations may possess abuse-deterrent qualities, with the inclusion of naloxone in combination sublingual tablets as the most well-known. Additionally, buprenorphine/naloxone sublingual film is more difficult to crush than the tablets, and is intended to discourage abuse [6]. If subdermal buprenorphine implants are eventually approved for use, this will provide another option in the arsenal of abuse deterrent formulations.

SAFETY

Buprenorphine is generally safe and well-tolerated, with an improved safety profile over full mu-agonists [2, 80]. Buprenorphine shares many adverse effects of typical opioids, but also causes unique pharmacologic effects worth noting. Indications, dosing information, and side effect profiles of various buprenorphine formulations are listed in Table 1, with additional discussion below.

Ceiling Effect and Respiratory Depression

As a partial mu-agonist, buprenorphine has a well-known ceiling for physiological and subjective effects [2, 81-83]. This effect is most likely due to pharmacodynamic, not pharmacokinetic, factors [84]. The plateau of effects for buprenorphine mitigates some risk for overdose, as there is low toxicity even at high doses used for the treatment of opioid dependence [24, 32, 80, 85].

It has been proposed that the ceiling in pharmacologic effect may limit abuse liability [24, 32]. However, Walsh *et al.* described euphoric and sedative effects of higher buprenorphine doses similar in magnitude to methadone 60 mg orally or morphine 30 mg IV, and abuse has been reported frequently [24].

Respiratory depression is the most dangerous adverse effect of opioids, mediated by mu receptors and caused by decreased sensitivity to carbon dioxide at chemoreceptors in the medulla oblongata [86]. Buprenorphine has the lowest incidence among opioids, but dose-dependent effects on respiration have been observed [31-32, 45, 87]. Intravenous administration may reduce mean respiratory rate and increase mean arterial carbon dioxide tension, with greater effects observed for 0.4 mg versus 0.2 mg [88]. Still, the impact of buprenorphine on respiratory effects is usually limited and clinically insignificant. In studies where drowsiness and the slope of the carbon dioxide response curve were observed, changes were minor or did not require medical intervention [32].

A ceiling effect for respiratory depression has been observed at high doses in animal studies [89-90]. Respiratory depression has not been induced at doses 1,000-fold higher than analgesic doses and a ceiling effect for respiratory depression occurred at lower doses than for analgesia. The net effect is a wider safety margin for buprenorphine compared to traditional opioids when buprenorphine is used in absence of other drugs [2, 36, 45, 81-82]. Norbuprenorphine exerts more respiratory depressive effects than buprenorphine with up to 10-fold increased potency mediated by mu receptor agonism [44, 89].

Norbuprenorphine requires a 50-fold greater concentration than analgesic doses to induce respiratory depression.

Table 1. Buprenorphine dosing and adverse effects [6, 8, 60, 64]

	Buprenex® Parenteral	Buprenorphine Sublingual Tablet	Buprenorphine/ Naloxone Sublingual Tablet	Suboxone® Sublingual Film	Zubzolv® Sublingual Tablet	Butrans® Transdermal
Schedule	III	III	III	III	III	III
Indications and Usage	Relief of moderate to severe pain.	Treatment of opioid dependence and preferred for induction. Prescription use is limited under the Drug Addiction Treatment Act.	Maintenance treatment of opioid dependence. Prescription use of this product is limited under the Drug Addiction Treatment Act.	Maintenance treatment of opioid dependence. Prescription use of this product is limited under the Drug Addiction Treatment Act.	Maintenance treatment of opioid dependence. Prescription use of this product is limited under the Drug Addiction Treatment Act.	Management of moderate to severe chronic pain in patients requiring continuous, around-the-clock opioid analgesic for an extended period of time. Not intended for PRN use, mild pain or pain expected to be short lasting, acute pain, postop pain (unless patient was receiving chronic opioid therapy prior to surgery or if postop pain is expected to be moderate to severe and persist for a long-term period).

	Buprenex® Parenteral	Buprenorphine Sublingual Tablet	Buprenorphine/ Naloxone Sublingual Tablet	Suboxone® Sublingual Film	Zubzolv® Sublingual Tablet	Butrans® Transdermal
Schedule	III	III	III	III	III	III
Dosage and Administration	13 years and older: 1 mL given by deep IM or slow (over at least 2 min) IV infusion at up to 6-hour intervals Children: 2-6 mcg/kg of body weight every 4-6 hours	SL as single daily dose. To avoid precipitating withdrawal, induction should begin when objective and clear signs of withdrawal are evident. Combinations containing naloxone are generally initiated after 2 days of buprenorphine titration.	Administer sublingually as a single daily dose. The recommended daily dose for maintenance is 16/4 mg.	Administer sublingually as a single daily dose. The recommended daily dose for maintenance treatment is 16 mg/4mg buprenorphine and naloxone. Advise patients not to cut, chew, or swallow sublingual film.	Administer sublingually as a single daily dose. The recommended daily dose for maintenance treatment is 11.4 mg /2.8 mg buprenorphine and naloxone. Advise patients not to cut, chew, or swallow.	Individualize dosing based on patient's prior analgesic experience, and titrate as needed to provide adequate analgesia and minimize adverse reactions. Wear patch for 7 days and wait a min of 3 weeks before applying to same site. Do not abruptly discontinue in a physically dependent patient.
Black Box Warnings	n/a	n/a	n/a	n/a	n/a	Abuse potential with liability similar to Schedule III opioids; life-threatening respiratory depression; accidental exposure, as exposure in children

Table 1. (Continued)

	Buprenex® Parenteral	Buprenorphine Sublingual Tablet	Buprenorphine/ Naloxone Sublingual Tablet	Suboxone® Sublingual Film	Zubzolv® Sublingual Tablet	Butrans® Transdermal
Schedule	III	III	III	III	III	III
						especially can result in fatal overdose.
Contraindications	Hypersensitivity to buprenorphine.	Hypersensitivity to buprenorphine.	Hypersensitivity to buprenorphine or naloxone.	Hypersensitivity to buprenorphine or naloxone.	Hypersensitivity to buprenorphine or naloxone.	Significant respiratory depression, acute or severe bronchial asthma. known or suspected paralytic ileus, hypersensitivity to buprenorphine.
Adverse effects	Most frequent side effect is sedation. Nausea and dizziness/vertigo.	Headache, nausea, vomiting, hyperhidrosis, constipation, withdrawal, insomnia, and pain.	Headache, nausea, vomiting, hyperhidrosis, constipation, signs and symptoms of withdrawal, insomnia, pain, and peripheral edema.	Oral hypoesthesia, glossodynia, oral mucosal erythema, headache, nausea, vomiting, hyperhidrosis, constipation, signs and symptoms of withdrawal, insomnia, pain, and peripheral edema.	Headache, nausea, vomiting, hyperhidrosis, constipation, signs and symptoms of withdrawal, insomnia, pain, and peripheral edema.	Nausea, headache, application site pruritus, dizziness, constipation, somnolence, vomiting, application site erythema, dry mouth, and application site rash.

Despite accumulation observed in chronic dosing, norbuprenorphine-induced respiratory depression is not common; minimal distribution into the CNS and a protective effect of buprenorphine appear to mitigate this risk [45, 86].

Use with concomitant CNS depressants such as benzodiazepines may alter the ceiling effect and increase the risk of respiratory depression (see Drug-Drug Interactions). The risk of respiratory depression is increased in elderly, cachectic, and debilitated patients due to altered pharmacokinetics resulting from poor fat stores, muscle wasting, and altered clearance. Patients with chronic obstructive pulmonary disease or cor pulmonale may also be at increased risk and should be monitored for apnea [6, 8]. Case reports of early respiratory depression following epidural administration have been published but these effects are rare, and at least some instances involved co-administration of other CNS-depressants including benzodiazepines [91]. Respiratory depression has resulted in fatal overdoses in some opioid naïve patients prior to reaching a ceiling, and this risk has been particularly noted in children (see Unintentional Exposures in Children) [92].

Opioid Antagonism

Due to partial mu agonism and high receptor affinity, buprenorphine may block the effects of exogenously administered opioids and precipitate abstinence syndrome in patients who are opioid dependent [2, 6, 13, 24, 93-95]. The magnitude of opioid antagonism is dependent on the dose of buprenorphine, the dose of the other opioid, and the time interval between administration [2, 20, 96-99]. Buprenorphine can displace opioids already administered, or ameliorate the effects of subsequent opioid doses for up to a day [15, 24, 93, 96, 98, 100]. Combinations of buprenorphine and other opioids may exert a synergistic effect when both are used at low doses, with mu receptor antagonism observed when high doses of buprenorphine or high doses of pure mu-agonists are used [20, 97-99, 101]. Buprenorphine-induced withdrawal is unlikely to occur with doses equivalent to or less than parenteral morphine 120 mg or oral methadone 30 mg [2, 97-98]. Likewise, buprenorphine 32 mg SL was more effective at producing opioid antagonism than the 2 mg SL dose [20]. Buprenorphine-induced antagonism may be overcome by higher doses of opioids, but this can complicate treatment when acute pain management is indicated [4, 93]. Nonetheless, the potential for antagonism of mu-agonists may be a desirable effect when buprenorphine is used for the treatment of opioid dependence in patients with a history of heroin or prescription opioid abuse [24].

Adverse Effects

Buprenorphine has the potential to induce hyperalgesia, which is opioid-induced nociceptive sensitization. Patients with hyperalgesia will develop paradoxical increases of pain as opioid doses are increased, an effect which has been more commonly described with pure mu-agonists [102]. Buprenorphine-induced hyperalgesia, demonstrated in animal models, appears to be mediated by the N-methyl-D-aspartate (NMDA) receptor [102-103]. Conflicting results have been reported in other animal studies wherein buprenorphine suppressed hyperalgesia by activation of the ORL-1 receptor, leading researchers to hypothesize that buprenorphine may have a role in the treatment of neuropathic pain [104]. Regardless, heroin abusers with hyperalgesia who are stabilized in methadone or buprenorphine maintenance treatment do not develop differences in pain responses, which would suggest that buprenorphine does not offer a substantial antihyperalgesic effect in this population [105].

The effect of buprenorphine on hepatic function has been investigated, as cytolytic hepatitis and jaundice have been observed in addicts receiving buprenorphine treatment for opioid dependence. Patients may be at risk for asymptomatic elevations in hepatic transaminases, hepatic failure, necrosis, hepato-renal syndrome, and encephalopathy [8]. The relative contribution of buprenorphine to these outcomes is unknown, as high rates of co-infection with hepatitis B or C, concurrent use with hepatotoxic drugs, and intravenous drug use in populations studied may be contributing factors [8, 80]. Baseline liver function tests are recommended prior to initiating treatment, with periodic monitoring thereafter [8]. In patients with hepatitis C, dosing of buprenorphine resulted in increased drug exposure with a 32% greater AUC. These findings suggest that patients with hepatitis C co-infection should be carefully monitored for both hepatic function and buprenorphine toxicity [106].

Sexual disturbances including erectile dysfunction, ejaculatory disturbances and decreased libido have been noted in patients on opioid therapy [107]. These effects are likely mediated by opioid-induced androgen deficiency (OPIAD), which results in lower testosterone levels and a host of other effects including fatigue and depression [108]. A meta-analysis indicates that lower testosterone levels are more common in patients maintained on methadone versus buprenorphine, with nearly twice the incidence of sexual dysfunction in users of methadone. While the lower incidence noted with buprenorphine may provide an advantage, sexual dysfunction has still been reported in 10% to 36% of patients and should be monitored accordingly [107].

Other adverse effects of buprenorphine which are typical of the opioid class include dizziness, headache, somnolence, insomnia, abdominal pain, constipation, nausea, vomiting, and hypotension. Less common reactions include spasm of the sphincter of Oddi, which may impact patients with biliary tract disease (e.g., pancreatitis). Buprenorphine is contraindicated in patients with paralytic ileus due to its potential to induce gastrointestinal dysfunction. Other severe effects include precipitation of seizures in patients with convulsive disorders and increased intracranial pressure. Hypersensitivity reactions may require rotation to a different opioid [6, 8].

There are unique safety considerations when initiating treatment with transdermal buprenorphine. Application site reactions including irritation, erythema, rash, and pruritus may be delayed by days or months. External heat or fever may increase absorption and can potentially cause fatal overdose; patients should be warned of this effect [8]. The safety of transdermal buprenorphine in patients under 18 years has not been established. The use of doses ranging from 8.75 to 140 mcg/hour administered every 3 days have been described in pediatric cancer patients, with small doses applied by cutting the patch into 2 or 4 pieces. These doses were administered using the Transtec® (Napp Pharmaceuticals, UK) 96-hour buprenorphine patch available in the United Kingdom [109]. The manufacturer of Butrans® cautions against cutting patches, but both Transtec® and Butrans® incorporate drug into an adhesive matrix which may allow for dosage adjustment by cutting (versus a drug reservoir type patch) [8, 110]. Bioequivalence of the buprenorphine patch has not been demonstrated in elderly patients (≥ 75 years) versus younger patients in the 50- to 60-year age group [111]. It has been proposed that a trend of higher concentrations of norbuprenorphine in elderly patients may be caused by decreased renal clearance [112]. However, similar tolerability for transdermal buprenorphine has been demonstrated between age groups [111, 113].

Labeling for transdermal buprenorphine also carries the unique warning for prolongation of the QTc interval, which can precipitate fatal cardiac arrhythmias such as torsades de pointes. Lengthening of the QT interval was noted with the buprenorphine 40 mcg/hour dose. Patients with hypokalemia or clinically unstable cardiac disease, a history of long QT syndrome or family member with the condition, or concurrent treatment with antiarrhythmic medications in Class IA (quinidine, procainamide, disopyramide) or Class III (sotalol, amiodarone, dofetilide), may have an increased risk [8]. The risk of buprenorphine-precipitated prolongation of QT intervals is lower than the risk with methadone, and several comparison studies have failed to note an effect of buprenorphine on the QT interval [31, 114-115]. Nevertheless, the manufacturer recommends a maximum dose of transdermal buprenorphine 20 mcg/hour to reduce this risk. Transdermal buprenorphine is also the only formulation with a black box warning, which advises of abuse potential liability similar to Schedule III opioids, life-threatening respiratory depression, and accidental exposure in children resulting in fatal overdose [8].

Lactation

Buprenorphine has been detected in breast milk for 2 hours following ingestion [116-117]. Both buprenorphine and norbuprenorphine have been detected in urine of breastfeeding infants. Exposure for breastfed infants may be low, with an infant buprenorphine dose per kg body weight under 1% of maternal dose [117]. Buprenorphine concentrations in breast milk are similar to maternal plasma concentrations [116-118]. Women receiving buprenorphine 4 mg/day excreted 3.3 mcg/day in breast milk; other studies have noted ranges of buprenorphine from 0.23 to 3.65 ng/mL, with norbuprenorphine 1.94 ng/mL detected in one case [118-120]. No adverse effects or signs of withdrawal have been noted up to 4 weeks in breastfed infants of mothers maintained on buprenorphine [31, 119-121]. Although breastfeeding patients taking buprenorphine can be reassured by these findings, infants should be monitored carefully [116-117, 120].

Withdrawal and Tolerance

Physical dependence may develop with prolonged buprenorphine administration, and abrupt discontinuation should be avoided [6, 8]. Physical dependence is not the same as the disease of addiction, but instead manifests as physiological adaptation which can produce withdrawal symptoms following discontinuation. Withdrawal symptoms include restlessness, lacrimation, rhinorrhea, yawning, perspiration, chills, myalgia, and mydriasis

[2, 8]. Withdrawal from buprenorphine causes symptoms of mild to moderate intensity compared to full mu-agonists, and some studies have demonstrated minimal or complete lack of symptoms following discontinuation of large doses up to 32 mg IM per day [2, 13, 96, 122-123]. Withdrawal may be minimized due to slow dissociation of buprenorphine from opioid receptors but generally follows the same time course as other opioids, with onset in 1 to 3 days, peak effect in 3 to 5 days, and an overall duration of 8 to 10 days [21, 124]. Inter-individual variability is likely, as some studies have found minimal symptoms occurring at 98 hours and delayed onset with symptoms peaking at 2 weeks in others [96, 125]. Brief interruptions in treatment should be well-tolerated with mild symptoms (if any should occur), as has been demonstrated by patients undergoing incarceration [126].

Tolerance develops to buprenorphine's pharmacologic effects, similar to other mu-agonists. Tolerance to behavioral and analgesic effects has been observed in animals, but appears to develop more slowly than tolerance to morphine [13, 127]. Cross-tolerance to the effects of other opioids has been demonstrated in animal studies [13, 67, 124].

Risk Evaluation and Mitigation Strategies (REMS)

Sublingual buprenorphine/naloxone is included in the FDA REMS program, which includes a medication guide, elements to ensure safe use (Dear Healthcare Provider letters, brochures, and appropriate use checklist), and an implementation system. The purpose of this program is to mitigate risk of accidental overdose, misuse, and abuse and inform prescribers, pharmacists, and patients of risks associated with buprenorphine-containing products. REMS programs are applicable when using sublingual buprenorphine for maintenance treatment, but not when used in patients admitted to a state-licensed opioid treatment facility under U.S. 42 CFR part 8 [60]. Several generic and brand sublingual products are enrolled in a shared program under the Buprenorphine-containing Transmucosal products of Opioid Dependence (BTOD) REMS [128]. The transdermal formulation of buprenorphine is included in the Extended-Release and Long-Acting (ER/LA) Opioid Analgesics REMS program, which also requires a medication guide, elements to ensure safe use, and assessments. The ER/LA REMS program is intended to reduce the risk of serious adverse outcomes resulting from inappropriate prescribing, misuse, and abuse of ER/LA opioid analgesics while maintaining patient access to pain medications [60].

Unintentional Exposures in Children

Unsupervised ingestion of buprenorphine by children is a concern, with an increasing number of cases reported by the Researched Abuse, Diversion, and Addiction-Related Surveillance System (RADARS) following the FDA approval of sublingual buprenorphine in 2002 [129-130]. Between October 2009 and March 2012, 2,380 cases of pediatric overdose in children less than 6 years old were reported to the RADARS Poison Center Program and Reckitt Benckiser Pharmaceuticals pharmacovigilance system [131]. From 2010 to 2011, the Centers for Disease Control and Prevention (CDC) estimates that 1,500 children less than 6 years old were evaluated in U.S. emergency departments (EDs) following accidental ingestion of buprenorphine products. During that same time period, buprenorphine was involved in about 30% of pediatric opioid-related ED visits and 59.5% of emergent hospitalizations for opioid product ingestion [130]. More than half of pediatric patients presenting to an ED with buprenorphine overdose required hospitalization and treatment in a pediatric intensive care unit (PICU) [92, 130]. Combination buprenorphine/naloxone tablets accounted for the largest proportion of toxic ingestions among children less than 3 years old admitted to a PICU [92].

Respiratory depression does not appear to have a ceiling effect in children and fatal overdoses have been reported [6, 131]. Postmortem concentrations of buprenorphine have been identified in serum in absence of other drugs, as buprenorphine alone appeared to cause death [132]. Buprenorphine can induce lethargy, respiratory depression, miosis, vomiting, agitation/irritability, pallor, and coma in children [92, 129, 131]. The onset of effects may occur in 1 hour, with duration of effects lasting 2 to 8 hours in 59% and 8 to 24 hours in 26% of children [129]. Because of the long duration of buprenorphine, continuous infusion of naloxone has been used in overdose management [92]. Naloxone may induce at least a partial response for two-thirds of patients, but is not always effective [129].

From 2002 through 2012, pediatric overdoses from buprenorphine/naloxone tablets have occurred far more frequently than the film product, with tablets identified in up to 96% exposures [129-131]. This increased risk for overdose through exposure to tablets may be due to the relatively recent FDA approval of the film in 2010 [65]. Transdermal systems contain between 5 mg to 20 mg buprenorphine per patch, depending on dose. Chewing of patches may pose a risk of exposure, and patches should be kept out of reach of children [8]. Buprenorphine has also been used in veterinary medicine as an injectable, oral spray, or liquid, which may also be a source of accidental ingestion [129]. Contributing factors associated with pediatric overdoses include storage of medications in sight, accessibility from a bag or purse, or storage in a container other than the original packaging [131]. In a case series of toddlers admitted to a PICU, all exposures occurred at home, though other cases have resulted from exposure by caretakers [92, 132]

Response to Naloxone

Buprenorphine's high affinity for mu receptors complicates treatment with naloxone, which has lower receptor affinity [22]. In a comparison of methadone, heroin, and buprenorphine overdoses, naloxone 0.4 to 0.8 mg was not effective at reversing mental status depression caused by buprenorphine. Co-ingestion of sedatives was frequent, occurring in 95% of buprenorphine overdoses. The investigators noted improvement with administration of flumazenil, a benzodiazepine antagonist, in cases involving ingestion of benzodiazepines [133]. Although these are typical doses for naloxone reversal of opioid overdose, reversal of buprenorphine may require doses 10 to 50 times greater than those used to reverse full mu-agonists, and doses up to 35 mg/70 kg have been described [2, 22, 91, 134]. In animal models, prophylactic naloxone 10 mg/kg IV blocked the analgesic effects of high-dose buprenorphine 0.68 mg/kg IV. Established buprenorphine agonism is less sensitive to naloxone reversal, though repeated naloxone doses may induce complete antagonism [99].

Naloxone typically reverses full mu-agonists within 2 minutes, but antagonism of buprenorphine may be delayed by 30 to 60 minutes with a maximum reversal effect noted at 3 hours [2, 8, 134]. Due to buprenorphine's long elimination half-life, its duration may exceed naloxone's (typically between 1 and 4 hours) by ten-fold [2, 13]. Repeated doses of naloxone, preferably by continuous infusion, are required in the management of buprenorphine overdose and monitoring should continue for at least 24 hours [2, 8, 45, 83]. In some cases, naloxone may not be effective even when high doses are used, which may suggest a non-opioid mechanism and a role of ORL-1 receptors in respiratory depression [2, 8, 11, 59].

Drug-Drug Interactions

Additive CNS/respiratory depression may be observed if buprenorphine is used in combination with other medications such as benzodiazepines, skeletal muscle relaxants, or other CNS depressants such as alcohol [6, 8]. Other medications noted to increase this risk include antidepressants, sedatives/anxiolytics including phenobarbital and zolpidem, phenothiazines, antipsychotics, and anticholinergics [8, 135]. Some animal studies have demonstrated a limited role for pharmacokinetic interactions with selected agents. For example, buprenorphine increased the AUC for desmethylflunitrazepam, the metabolite of the benzodiazepine flunitrazepam, which could have a potential role in toxicity [136]. Additionally, midazolam moderately inhibits CYP3A4 metabolism of buprenorphine to norbuprenorphine [137]. However, the clinical significance of these interactions in unknown, and the majority of interactions appear to be pharmacodynamic rather than pharmacokinetic [138].

Benzodiazepines

Caution is recommended when using buprenorphine and benzodiazepines concomitantly [6]. Animal studies have demonstrated respiratory depressant effects with the co-administration of benzodiazepines; despite minimal effects when these agents are used alone, profound synergistic effects are noted when they are used together [139-140]. Monotherapy with buprenorphine typically results in a bell-shaped dose response curve for respiratory depression. The protective ceiling effect is eliminated with co-administration of other CNS depressants, especially in the presence of supratherapeutic doses of benzodiazepines [141-142]. In a human study of buprenorphine and diazepam administered at therapeutic doses, marked respiratory effects did not occur; consequently it has been suggested that therapeutic use of benzodiazepines are less concerning than doses exceeding recommended guidelines [143].

The strength of the interactions may vary depending not only on dose, but also the selected benzodiazepine. Flunitrazepam and midazolam have been implicated as likely candidates to induce respiratory effects in animal studies; although international reports of overdose have occurred, these drugs are rarely used in the outpatient setting in the U.S. [59, 140]. Despite these findings, toxicological analysis has revealed a broad range of benzodiazepines identified in fatal overdoses. Diazepam has been the most common identified drug in multiple international reports [135, 142, 144-147]. Other benzodiazepines identified in medical examiner reports include alprazolam, bromazepam, clorazepate, flunitrazepam, midazolam, nitrazepam, oxazepam, and temazepam [2, 59, 135, 142, 147-148]. These reports suggest a limited correlation of toxicity to dose-dependent effects, as concentrations of benzodiazepines have been reported in the therapeutic range despite fatal outcome [142, 147]. The most frequently used benzodiazepines in the U.S. are (in order), diazepam, alprazolam, lorazepam, and clonazepam, and all have been implicated in dangerous or fatal overdoses when ingested with buprenorphine [59, 135, 142, 144-147, 149-151]. Patients participating in buprenorphine maintenance who are prescribed benzodiazepines are more frequently involved in ED visits than those without a benzodiazepine prescription [152]. Despite this risk, benzodiazepines may be frequently used for anxiety or withdrawal symptoms for patients also prescribed buprenorphine [153]. Some practitioners recommend avoiding benzodiazepines in opioid treatment programs, as they may limit the development of psychological coping mechanisms or impair efficacy of cognitive-behavioral therapy [154-155]. Controversy exists over the contribution of benzodiazepine use to relapse, with some evidence supporting a correlation between benzodiazepine and cocaine/opiate use [156-157]. Other studies demonstrate no significant differences in clinical outcomes for treatment retention or illicit opioid/cocaine use, with or without benzodiazepines [152]. It may be that patients using benzodiazepines, whether licit or illicit, have a more complicated clinical picture which may impede the treatment for opioid dependence. Regardless, benzodiazepine misuse can pose a significant safety concern in a population at risk for drug abuse [158-159]. Given these concerns, experts have recommended benzodiazepines only as maintenance therapy for patients with benzodiazepine dependence or for the treatment of severe anxiety disorders, with antidepressants such as selective serotonin reuptake inhibitors (SSRIs) or serotonin-norepinephrine reuptake inhibitors (SNRIs) used as first-line treatment for anxiety. If benzodiazepines must be used as adjunctive therapy, use should be short-term with scheduled dosing, and a long-acting benzodiazepine may be preferred [152, 160].

CYP3A4 Inhibitors or Inducers

CYP3A4 inhibitors and inducers may affect buprenorphine pharmacokinetics and necessitate monitoring, though the clinical impact of such interactions is often unclear [6]. Interactions with antiretrovirals have been studied *in vivo*, with buprenorphine pharmacokinetic alterations noted via CYP3A4/5 and CYP2C8 [49]. *In vitro* data suggests that ritonavir could result in complete inhibition of CYP3A4 metabolism of buprenorphine to norbuprenorphine, with significant inhibition by indinavir as well. Use of protease inhibitors may result in increased buprenorphine exposure, which could necessitate dosage adjustments [31]. Most antiretrovirals do not cause buprenorphine withdrawal or toxicity with exception of atazanavir/ritonavir, which can contribute to adverse effects such CNS depression/sedation [95]. CYP3A4 induction by efavirenz, nevirapine, and etravirine and inhibition by delavirdine are possible, but have not been shown to have significant pharmacodynamic effects for patients taking buprenorphine [6]. Further research is needed for antiretrovirals, though it appears there are fewer impactful drug-drug interactions with buprenorphine than for methadone [95].

Ketoconazole/indole derivatives may inhibit CYP3A4 and increase exposure to buprenorphine [31]. The degree of inhibition is dependent on both dose and duration, with maximal inhibition observed for ketoconazole 400 mg/day administered for several days. More frequent dosing (twice daily versus once daily) can lead to a greater degree of inhibition. However, ketoconazole 200 mg BID did not increase exposure of transdermal buprenorphine 10 mcg/hour, probably due to lack of first-pass hepatic and intestinal metabolism via the transdermal route. Increased exposure to sublingual buprenorphine (up to 2-fold) occurs when administered with ketoconazole; investigators theorized that impaired first-pass metabolism increased bioavailability of the portion of the tablet that is swallowed [161]. Consequently, the route of administration may be an important variable to consider when evaluating potential drug-drug interactions.

Other potential interactions include CYP3A4 inhibition by SSRI antidepressants, particularly with norfluoxetine (a metabolite of fluoxetine) and fluvoxamine. Anticonvulsants including phenobarbital, carbamazepine, and phenytoin can induce CYP3A4, thereby lowering buprenorphine concentrations.

Rifampin is a potent CYP3A4 inducer which can reduce buprenorphine exposure, and experts have recommended avoiding concurrent use with buprenorphine [4, 31]. *In vitro* studies indicate that buprenorphine is a strong inhibitor of CYP3A4 and CYP2D6. Weak inhibition of CYP1A2, CYP2B6, CYP2C19, CYP2C8, CYP2E1, and CYP2A6 may be possible; *in vivo*, therapeutic concentrations are sufficiently low that interactions are not clinically significant [45].

ADDICTION/OPIOID DEPENDENCE

Opioid abuse has increased significantly during the last decade. In 2012, more than 2 million people in the U.S. reported nonmedical use of prescription pain relievers [162]. Opioid-related overdoses have been called an epidemic by the CDC, with one unintentional death occurring every 19 minutes [163]. Opioid abuse is also extremely costly, with prescription opioid dependence resulting in $55.7 billion in societal costs [164]. Current spending on addiction research and prevention is minimal in comparison. Methadone has been used for more than 40 years for the treatment of opioid dependence and is the predominant treatment in the U.S., where it is administered in once daily doses in highly regulated settings [165-166]. Heroin abuse is presently at the highest rate since the 1970s, and yet is dwarfed by the 3-fold higher prevalence of prescription opioid abuse [162]. Despite the increasing need for treatment of opioid dependence, methadone maintenance programs have not kept pace [94].

Buprenorphine treatment for opioid dependence was introduced internationally in 1980 and has been safely used to withdraw patients from heroin and prescription opioids [3, 167-169]. Like methadone, buprenorphine may be used either as long-term opioid substitution therapy, or as short-term treatment with eventual detoxification. Craving scores typically plateau at 2 weeks after initiation of buprenorphine, thus reducing illicit drug use [170]. Buprenorphine offers a substantial improvement over adrenergic agonists in its side effect profile and the management of opioid withdrawal symptoms [171]. It has a good long-term safety profile and has been used in maintenance therapy for up to 5 years with no serious adverse effects [172]. In 2007, both buprenorphine and buprenorphine/naloxone formulations were added to the 15th World Health Organization Model List of Essential Medicines [4].

Many studies have demonstrated similar efficacy between methadone and buprenorphine, though comparisons have found varying results across different dosages [167-169, 173-176]. Buprenorphine may cause less rewarding effects and sedation than methadone. Some users may seek only to decrease use rather than discontinue illicit opioids, and buprenorphine's blocking effects at mu receptors may limit treatment retention. Other patients may object to the taste of buprenorphine or the time required for the sublingual preparations to dissolve [177]. Patient preference may influence provider choice of buprenorphine or methadone, with buprenorphine most likely selected for short-term detoxification and methadone for long-term maintenance [178].

The World Health Organization (WHO) recommends methadone for most patients on the basis of clinical efficacy and decreased cost. However, the WHO also recommends that both methadone and buprenorphine be made available as treatment options for opioid maintenance and withdrawal. Methadone programs may bear a social stigma, and nearly a third of patients who seek treatment with buprenorphine would not have presented to a methadone-based opioid treatment program [177, 179]. Regardless of which treatment is selected, desirable outcomes such as treatment retention and abstinence from illicit/opioid use are highly variable, and multi-modal therapy should include inpatient or outpatient counseling [180].

High doses of sublingual buprenorphine 1 to 32 mg/day are used for the treatment of opioid dependence [181]. The buprenorphine mono-product is most often used for induction to reduce the chance of withdrawal from the full mu-agonist opioid, though buprenorphine/naloxone may also be used [3, 94, 101]. Suppression of withdrawal is dose-dependent, and lower doses during the induction phase are associated with continued opioid use [182-185]. Withdrawal may be noted at start of therapy as buprenorphine may not completely substitute for the full mu-agonist [167, 186]. Some studies have demonstrated the occurrence of increased withdrawal symptoms when lower buprenorphine doses are used, while others have found more withdrawal with higher buprenorphine doses; the outcome depends on time course following the full mu-agonist, the level of opioid dependence, and the type of opioid used (e.g., long- or short-acting). Prescribers initiating buprenorphine induction therapy must strike a difficult balance between the effects of the full mu-agonist, the agonist-antagonist effects of buprenorphine, and the clinical state of the patient. Ideally, the patient should be exhibiting some signs of opioid withdrawal prior to initiating induction [98, 101]. Buprenorphine 4 mg SL may be used as a starting dose and increased over several days until the patient is stabilized over 24 hours, which will usually necessitate a target dose between 8 mg to 24 mg daily [179]. Buprenorphine's long duration of action allows for once daily dosing, but less than daily dosing has been used in some studies, with regimens of 8 mg to 32 mg every other day or 16 mg to 32 mg three times per week. Withdrawal symptoms may be absent or minimal with less-frequent dosing regimens [21, 24, 98, 123, 176, 179, 187-190]. Alternate day dosing has been used for over two decades in some programs [3]. Supervised dosing is recommended in the early phase of treatment and should be considered on an individual basis thereafter [179]. Less frequent dosing may be useful in these circumstances, particularly as flexibility is important for patients under supervision [191]. Such dosing regimens may also be beneficial and can be enacted under observed conditions if diversion is suspected [101].

Outcomes

Evidence from multiple studies demonstrates that a significant number of patients enrolled in buprenorphine maintenance therapy will discontinue treatment. Retention rates are higher for buprenorphine at doses greater than 2 mg/day than for placebo [192]. Buprenorphine used in flexible or low doses is less effective than methadone in ensuring patient retention (relative risk 0.83) [192-193]. Treatment retention and abstinence from illicit use do not differ for patients taking buprenorphine 16 to 32 mg/day versus methadone, with this dosage range of buprenorphine predicting better retention than lower doses of buprenorphine [114, 175, 192]. Retention rates reported in studies at the end of treatment with buprenorphine range from 4 to 100%, with a median of 66% [194]. Retention may be quite low even for patients who have been previously stable; of patients who had already been stable in treatment for 6 months, retention at 2 years was only 38% [172]. Patients actively enrolled in maintenance treatment may or may not be compliant with prescribed treatment. Weeks of compliance, defined as detection of buprenorphine on urine drug test (UDT) results during buprenorphine maintenance, has been demonstrated between 74 to 95% [195]. Despite moderate levels of success in keeping patients in treatment, buprenorphine maintenance outperforms attempts to taper or detoxify patients (see section on "Detoxification") [172].

It is to be expected that some patients will persist in positive UDT findings for opioids and illicit drugs, as rates of continued use are fairly high [185]. Comparisons of patients retained in buprenorphine and methadone maintenance indicate no difference in outcomes for abstinence, and opioids or illicit drugs are detected in 34% to 69% of urine specimens [153, 169, 187, 192, 195-200]. The median number of patients in treatment with non-adherent opioid-positive specimens is 59% [194]. Notably, only high dose buprenorphine ≥16 mg performs better than placebo in suppressing illicit use shown by UDT [192]. Patients stabilized on buprenorphine maintenance for 2 to 5 years may have higher rates of abstinence, with only 9% of patients testing positive for illicits/opioids [172].

Multiple factors may affect treatment outcome for patients maintained with buprenorphine for opioid dependence. Components of a patient's medical history that are predictive of drug use during or after treatment include high level of opioid use pre-treatment, prior treatment for opioid addiction, no prior abstinence from opioids, abstinence from or light use of alcohol, comorbid anxiety disorders, active benzodiazepine use, and depression. Predictive environmental and social factors include high stress, unemployment, and association with drug-using peers. Short length of treatment, discontinuation prior to treatment completion, and high maintenance dose are associated with illicit drug use as well. No single factor is strongly predictive for treatment outcome [201-202]. Associations with some factors have not been confirmed in other studies, as some investigators have not established a link between historical or current benzodiazepine use and relapse [152]. Continued opioid abuse and uncontrolled pain are both predictors for dropping out of buprenorphine maintenance treatment; pain does not have the same impact on retention rates for patients maintained on methadone [114, 203]. Finally, differences in the type of opioid misuse may influence treatment outcomes, with patients dependent on prescription opiates demonstrating higher treatment adherence and lower relapse rates than patients with a history of heroin abuse [204-205]. Demographic data such as gender and education have no relationship with continued illicit or opioid use [201].

Even in patients who do not achieve complete opioid or illicit drug abstinence, buprenorphine treatment may be advantageous in reducing harm. Depressing the amount of intravenous drug abuse or high-risk behaviors may prevent the spread of human immunodeficiency (HIV) or hepatitis C viruses, decrease morbidity and mortality, improve psychosocial functioning, and reduce criminal activity [3, 27, 179, 206-208]. Buprenorphine treatment may yield economic benefits as well. Opioid-dependent patients and abusers enrolled in buprenorphine maintenance for over one year had lower overall healthcare costs compared to patients with evidence suggestive of opioid misuse (adjusted means: $21,492 vs $47,868) [209].

Implementation

Since its established utility for the treatment of opioid dependence, buprenorphine has been adopted in treatment programs around the world. In many countries such as France and Germany, buprenorphine was approved earlier than in the U.S. [3, 135, 210]. Some countries initially only used the buprenorphine mono-product with few regulations governing its use. The introduction of the buprenorphine/naloxone combination product and stricter rules regarding prescribing and dispensing were subsequently enacted in effort to curtail burgeoning reports of misuse and abuse. International practices vary widely. In Australia, where buprenorphine has been used for opioid dependence since 2000, patients frequently receive supervised doses in a clinic or pharmacy [3]. Approximately one quarter of cases in Europe are currently addressed with buprenorphine, while the majority of patients are enrolled in methadone maintenance [210]. In France, buprenorphine is the predominant treatment for opioid dependence with few barriers from regulatory restrictions [2, 211]. All primary care physicians have the option to prescribe buprenorphine for opioid dependence, and no specific training or limit to the number of patients is required [3]. Additionally, pharmacists in France may dispense buprenorphine and supervise ingestion. Economic access is ensured as opioid dependence is considered a chronic illness, allowing full coverage by social security [211]. The adoption of buprenorphine treatment for opioid dependence has reduced rates of HIV among injection users, and decreased overdose deaths from heroin and cocaine by 80% from 1996 to 2003 [3, 211-212]. The successful reduction of opioid mortality rates in France is a case study supporting fewer restrictions to buprenorphine access and treatment [211].

Implementation of buprenorphine for the treatment of opioid dependence in the U.S. has been slower to take hold. FDA approval of the sublingual formulations in 2002 allowed treatment in an office-based setting for the first time, which in turn minimized contact with other drug users and reduced the stigma of drug dependence [3, 213]. The Drug Addiction Treatment Act of 2000 (DATA 2000) was enacted to allow physician certification for prescribing buprenorphine once certain requirements were met. Physicians must undergo training and obtain a waiver from the requirement to register as a narcotic treatment program from the Center for Substance Abuse Treatment (CSAT) of the Substance Abuse and Mental Health Services Administration [94]. Initially, physicians could treat no more than 30 patients in their practice at a time, but this limit was increased to 100 in 2006 [5]. Availability is still limited in the U.S. more than a decade later, with less than one third of substance abuse treatment programs offering maintenance with buprenorphine [166].

Availability is typically restricted to urban, highly populated areas and to patients with insurance plans, and not all patients have equal access to treatment with buprenorphine [214]. Despite these barriers, the favorable safety profile of buprenorphine led the U.S. National Institute on Drug Abuse to recommend buprenorphine as a first-line treatment for opioid dependence [3].

Use in Pregnancy

Exposure to illicit drugs in pregnancy can cause low birth weight or premature birth [116, 215-220]. While the treatment of opioid dependence is of critical importance during pregnancy, the choice of agent is controversial. In the U.S., methadone has been the only drug recommended in this setting although there is increasing evidence of a role for buprenorphine [4, 94, 221]. Likewise, the WHO recommends methadone over buprenorphine due to less available safety data for the latter, but sanctions buprenorphine as an option [179]. Experts have expressed concern for precipitation of opioid withdrawal and resulting deleterious effects in the fetus, especially with formulations containing naloxone [220]. For this reason, all patients in Finland receive buprenorphine/naloxone except pregnant women, who receive only the buprenorphine mono-product [222]. Maternal outcomes following use of buprenorphine or buprenorphine/naloxone appear to be similar to methadone [220].

Buprenorphine disposition may be altered in pregnant women due to changes in bioavailability and clearance. Increases in cardiac output (up to 30%), renal clearance, blood volume (up to 50%), and total body water (8 L) have been described [223-225]. Drug-protein binding may be reduced secondary to decreases in serum albumin concentrations and increases in steroids and placental hormones [223]. Metabolism via CYP3A4, CYP2D6, and CYP2C9 and some UGT enzymes may increase, while CYP1A2 and CYP2C19 activity may decrease [226]. These metabolic changes may necessitate dose adjustment throughout or during later stages of pregnancy [116, 225].

There do not appear to be significant effects of buprenorphine *in utero*, though some changes have been described [116, 227]. The amount of drug transfer to the infant depends on absorption from the gastrointestinal tract, extraction in liver, lipid solubility, protein binding, and molecular weight [117]. Though fetal buprenorphine exposure does occur, it is limited compared to maternal plasma concentrations [228]. Research indicates inhibition of CYP19/aromatase, a key enzyme for the biosynthesis of estrogens in the human placenta, by buprenorphine and to a lesser extent, norbuprenorphine. The placenta is the major source of 17β-estradiol (E_2), estriol (E_3), and estrone in maternal and fetal circulation. These estrogens regulate placental functions and progesterone biosynthesis, and low concentrations of estriol have been noted to correlate with low fetal and placental weight. Given these concerns, some experts suggest monitoring estrogen levels in pregnancy [229].

CYP19/aromatase can also be inhibited by methadone, though not as effectively as buprenorphine. Other opioids have this capability as well, and although acute use is unlikely to cause long-term effects, the implications of chronic use are unclear. To date, there are no reports in the clinical population [229-230]. The majority of infants born to mothers maintained on buprenorphine are full-term with normal birth parameters. Occasional cases of intrauterine growth restriction, preterm delivery, or sudden infant death syndrome (SIDS) are described; however, causation cannot be determined, as ongoing maternal use of illicit drugs or nicotine are frequently occurring confounding variables which could also be responsible [116, 219-220, 231]. Reported frequencies of malformations for infants of mothers treated with buprenorphine are not different than for methadone, even when high doses are used [218, 232]. Overall, buprenorphine appears to have an improved fetal safety profile over methadone. Buprenorphine causes less physiological suppression of fetal heart rate and movements, and potentially results in increases in gestational age at birth and birth weight [4, 116, 233]. There is no significant correlation between maternal buprenorphine dose and birth weight, gestational age at delivery, Apgar scores at 1 and 5 min, neonatal head circumference, or length [231, 234]. These findings suggest a lack of evidence to support limiting buprenorphine dose to minimize neonatal effects, but more research is needed [234]. The effect of buprenorphine in improving fetal outcomes by reducing illicit use is apparent in France, where a 3-fold reduction in premature infants coincided with the advent of buprenorphine treatment from 1995 to 2003 [235].

Neonatal Abstinence Syndrome (NAS)

Opioid use during pregnancy may cause fetal exposure and physical dependence, resulting in neonatal abstinence syndrome (NAS) following birth. Because of widespread use and abuse of prescription opioids, the incidence of NAS is a growing concern. From 2000 to 2009, cases of NAS in the U.S. increased from 1.2 to 3.4 per 1000 hospital live births [234]. Many cases require treatment in a neonatal intensive care unit [219]. Unlike opioid withdrawal in adults, NAS may be life threatening for infants [8]. Rates of treatment for NAS for infants of mothers maintained on buprenorphine have varied between 0% to 100%, with an average of 44% to 48% [116, 216, 219-22, 231, 233]. The development of NAS symptoms can be confounded by maternal use of additional drugs, as rates of concomitant ingestion of illicit drugs or nicotine may be high [216, 231].

Buprenorphine-associated NAS may last for 120 to 168 hours, with a mean time to onset of 53 hours and peak symptoms between 72 and 96 hours [116, 216]. Exceptions to this time frame may occur with delayed onset of NAS occurring on days 8 to 10, particularly if withdrawal to other medications such as benzodiazepines is present [116]. Delayed onset may have clinical significance; if maternal buprenorphine use is not recognized by the treating clinician, both mother and infant may be discharged from the delivering hospital prior to onset of symptoms. NAS from buprenorphine is less severe than methadone and fewer infants will require treatment [31, 116, 118, 211, 216, 232-233, 236-238]. For those infants undergoing treatment, withdrawal from methadone required treatment 12 hours earlier than buprenorphine-associated NAS [239]. Lower doses of substitutive treatment are usually needed for infants with buprenorphine-associated NAS, with doses up to three times higher recorded for infants withdrawing from methadone [233, 236, 240]. Treatment duration is shorter for buprenorphine cases (4.1 days versus 9.9 days for methadone), and ranges from 4.9 to 9.7 days [116, 220, 233, 240]. These benefits have resulted in statistically significant shorter hospital stays ranging from 4.7 to 37 days (mean 21.3 days) [116, 233, 240-241]. The overall duration of hospital stays for infants of buprenorphine-maintained mothers ranges from 4 to 27.3 days, with a mean of 14.7 days; breastfeeding is associated with shorter stays [116, 220, 240-241]. There is a lack of relationship between maternal dose at delivery and NAS severity, need for NAS treatment, duration of treatment, or duration of hospital stay [218, 231, 233-234, 239, 241, 243]. The overall favorable profile of buprenorphine compared to methadone may make it a useful treatment option for pregnant women, though the risk of NAS should be recognized.

DETOXIFICATION

Some patients may prefer detoxification to extended maintenance with buprenorphine [244-247]. In one study, 28% of patients desired treatment less than 6 months, and 42% left treatment within that time frame. The most common reasons for leaving treatment given by patients were conflict with staff, involuntary discharge, and a perception of inflexibility in the program [248]. Others may desire short-term treatment due to limited access to maintenance programs, especially in rural areas [249-252]. Patient selection for detoxification programs may be imperative for minimizing poor outcomes. Patients more likely to have a favorable response include those with demographic or drug use characteristics suggestive of low baseline severity of dependence/abuse, including non-injecting drug users and those with greater social stability [253-257].

Withdrawal symptoms during tapered detoxification may be diminished by buprenorphine's long duration of action and slow dissociation from opioid receptors [21, 188]. This benefit of buprenorphine may permit accelerated taper schedules to be used; however, most findings indicate that a taper is preferred over abrupt cessation [21, 213]. The duration of buprenorphine detoxification programs may vary from 0 days (abrupt discontinuation) to 120 days, with a median of 17 days. Taper duration is a predictor of relapse at the end of treatment as measured by opioid positive UDT results, but a stronger relationship has been demonstrated for days spent in maintenance [194, 213]. Longer tapers are associated with higher rates of opioid abstinence for both methadone and buprenorphine [21,188, 205, 258-262]. Some experts have recommended using gradual dose reductions interspersed with stabilization periods [261]. Other detoxification programs have used the 7-day transdermal patch, adjunct treatment with gabapentin, or increased buprenorphine dose of 32 mg prior to initiating a taper [3, 123, 263]. The WHO cautions against accelerated taper schedules in combination with sedation due to safety concerns [179].

Although withdrawal symptoms may be low during detoxification, relapse rates may still be poor [264]. Success rates between 2.5% and 13% have been described for methadone maintenance treatment in more than 14,000 episodes of detoxification [261]. Opioid abstinence rates demonstrated on UDT at the end of the taper have ranged from 22% to 63% [194, 213, 262]. Unfortunately, rates of opioid abstinence are typically lower at follow-up [194]. For subjects who have undergone detoxification in the previous 4 weeks to 24 months, opioid abstinence was noted in only 7 to 29% of patients [205, 213, 259, 264-265]. Ling *et al.* cautioned that prolonging tapers may not provide benefit; although rates of relapse were higher immediately following a 7-day versus a 28-day taper, outcomes were not significantly different in the long-term [213]. Poor outcomes have been consistently demonstrated in studies of detoxification, both with and without counseling [205]. The chronicity of addiction, combined with the dearth of effective strategies patients may use to prevent relapse, may undermine detoxification success. In many cases, maintenance therapy for long-term treatment may be preferable [244, 205, 259, 265-266].

PAIN MANAGEMENT

Buprenorphine has been used for more than 40 years as an analgesic. Its efficacy, tolerability, and safety have made it a useful adjunct for anesthesia, and acute and chronic pain [2-3]. It has been widely prescribed for pain management in Europe since the early 1980s, whereas its limited availability as an injectable product resulted in sparing use in the U.S. [267]. To date, transdermal buprenorphine is the only formulation in the U.S. with an indication for moderate to severe chronic pain, though sublingual buprenorphine products have been used off-label for this purpose [8, 100]. Use of buprenorphine/naloxone for pain management is not prohibited by DATA; nevertheless, practitioners may wish to adhere to DATA requirements when prescribing sublingual buprenorphine for pain, particularly if there is ambiguity regarding elements of physical dependence and therapeutic intent may be misinterpreted [100, 181].

Lower doses of buprenorphine are used for pain management than those used in the treatment of opioid dependence, and typically range from 0.1 to 0.8 mg/day [78, 181]. There is no published data to suggest a maximum analgesic dose in humans, and higher doses up to 10 mg/day have been used to elicit an analgesic response [2, 100]. Parenteral buprenorphine 0.3 mg is approximately equivalent to intramuscular morphine 10 mg [2]. Buprenorphine administered intramuscularly is approximately twice as potent as the sublingual route [268]. Opioid rotation and calculation of equianalgesic doses may be highly individualized, particularly at high doses due to the nonlinear mu agonism dose-response curve [11, 269-270].

Sublingual buprenorphine exerts a longer duration of action than intramuscular administration or morphine, but its analgesic effect lasts approximately 6 to 8 hours, thus requiring dosing 3 to 4 times per day [100, 268]. Experts have suggested rotating to a full mu-agonist if pain is not controlled by sublingual buprenorphine 32 mg/day [100]. Transdermal buprenorphine may be useful for patients who cannot take oral medications, such as patients with refractory nausea and vomiting, or cancer patients with head, neck, mouth, or bowel lesions [2]. Dosing titration for transdermal administration occurs very slowly. An initial dose increase of 5 mcg/hour may be made after 7 days, and every 72 hours thereafter up to a maximum of 20 mcg/hour. This can impair effective treatment for patients with rapidly changing analgesic requirements, particularly if high doses are required [271].

Buprenorphine has been administered via the epidural route in doses of 0.06 to 0.15 mcg, which can provide analgesia for 6 to 24 hours. Higher doses of 0.3 to 0.9 have also been described, but with little additional benefit [2, 91]. Intrathecal doses of 0.03 to 0.045 mg may also be administered with bupivacaine [2]. The mean time to the first request for postoperative analgesia was longer for patients receiving intrathecal buprenorphine versus dexmedetomidine, with a median sedation score lower for patients in the buprenorphine group; both effects were statistically significant [272]. These results suggest a role for buprenorphine in neuraxial dosing. Patient-controlled administration by the sublingual, intravenous, and intramuscular routes have been used, and subcutaneous buprenorphine may be delivered by implanted micropumps or continuous infusion [2].

Buprenorphine may be an effective option for acute pain, providing similar pain relief to full mu-agonists while potentially sparing some of the sedative and respiratory depressive effects. One study indicated patients receiving sublingual buprenorphine were more conscious in the immediate postoperative period than patients receiving intramuscular buprenorphine or meperidine [273]. Sublingual buprenorphine 2 mg has also been compared to intravenous morphine for use in acute renal colic; pain scores did not differ significantly, and adverse effects were similar despite more dizziness reported in patients receiving buprenorphine [274]. Buprenorphine has also been used successfully for chronic pain, particularly in patients also at risk for addiction or with opioid dependence [4, 181].

Despite moderate analgesia, buprenorphine may provide quality of life benefits; improvement in activities of daily living was noted following 12 weeks of transdermal buprenorphine use in patients with chronic low back pain [4, 271]. However, given the antagonism effects on other opioids and analgesic ceiling, buprenorphine is typically considered a second-line agent. Studies of patients using transdermal buprenorphine have indicated a high rate of discontinuation due to inadequate pain relief and side effects [4]. Cancer pain in particular may prove to be difficult to manage with buprenorphine in patients with very high analgesic requirements [2]. An observational study of patients converting from full mu-agonist opioids to sublingual buprenorphine indicated greater reductions in pain for patients taking lower doses of morphine equivalents (100-199 mg/day) versus higher dose equivalents (>400 mg/day) [103]. Conversely, a small study of cancer patients receiving between 150 to 516 mg morphine/day rotating to transdermal buprenorphine demonstrated no difference in pain before or after switching [270]. Individual response to buprenorphine may vary, but practitioners must be mindful that rotation to full mu-agonists may be required.

The antagonist effects of buprenorphine on other opioids may present a unique challenge in the setting of acute and postoperative pain. If a patient undergoing buprenorphine treatment experiences mild pain, buprenorphine titration may provide acceptable analgesia. Practitioners must expect a blunted analgesic response should other opioids be required, and breakthrough pain may require a high potency opioid such as fentanyl or hydromorphone at higher than normal doses [93, 100]. Patients should be carefully monitored during titration, as unexpected mu receptor sensitivity may occur with the gradual dissociation of buprenorphine [100]. If adjunctive opioids do not control pain, buprenorphine may be discontinued and restarted if pain resolves [94]. Patients should discontinue buprenorphine at least 72 hours before surgery, but may still require significantly increased doses of opioids during the postoperative period [4, 275]. Unexpected acute pain episodes may be undertreated for patients taking buprenorphine, particularly if practitioners are unfamiliar with buprenorphine's pharmacodynamic effects and necessity of elevated doses of opioids to overcome mu receptor antagonism.

PRESCRIPTION RATES

Buprenorphine implementation in the U.S. has lagged behind some European countries. Nonetheless, notable increases in buprenorphine availability have occurred during the past decade. The number of providers certified to prescribe buprenorphine for opioid dependence increased from 5,656 in 2005 to 18,582 in 2010 [276]. The advantage of office-based access has helped adoption in some states; in Utah for example, the number of buprenorphine prescribers increased 6,700% from 2002 to 2011 [277]. The use of buprenorphine in opioid treatment programs has seen a more modest increase, with the number of substance abuse treatment facilities offering buprenorphine increasing 231% from 2003 to 2010 [276]. Buprenorphine use has risen primarily for maintenance relative to detoxification. To date, 40% of opioid treatment programs in the U.S. still do not offer buprenorphine as an option [166]. In contrast, it has been adopted as the primary treatment in several countries internationally, including France, Finland, Sweden, Greece, Cyprus, and the Czech Republic [278].

Prescription rates in the U.S. have increased since sublingual buprenorphine was approved in 2002, with most attributed to treatment of opioid dependence and a limited proportion for pain management. According to the Drug Abuse Warning Network (DAWN), the number of patients prescribed buprenorphine increased from 100,000 in 2005 to 800,000 in 2010 [276]. In 2005, 8 million tablets were sold. By 2009, this figure had leapt to 145 million [279]. Similarly, 270,000 prescriptions were dispensed for sublingual buprenorphine in 2004, up to 9.3 million prescriptions in 2012 [5, 151]. The number of prescriptions dispensed for the buprenorphine/naloxone combination product is 12-fold higher than the buprenorphine mono-product, and the 8 mg/2 mg strength accounts for more than three quarters of dispensations [151]. Buprenorphine has held a place in the top 200 list of prescriptions for the past four years for which data is available, jumping from 189th in 2009 to 111th in 2012 [280-283]. In 2012, the only opioids that exceeded buprenorphine in number of prescriptions were hydrocodone, oxycodone, and tramadol; the only opioid that exceeded dollars spent on Suboxone® was OxyContin® (Purdue Pharma, U.S.) [283].

Abuse/Misuse

Buprenorphine has abuse liability similar to the mixed agonist-antagonist opioids such as pentazocine, butorphanol, and nalbuphine, with self-administration observed in early animal models [2, 127, 284]. In discrimination studies, subjects frequently identified buprenorphine as hydromorphone-like when asked to differentiate between administration of buprenorphine, hydromorphone, and placebo [285]. When compared to hydromorphone and pentazocine, patients identified buprenorphine as hydromorphone-like about half the time [286]. In essence, patients will identify buprenorphine as a mu-agonist if that is the only choice, but if exposed to mixed agonists-antagonists, buprenorphine classification falls somewhere in between the two.

The addition of naloxone does not completely eliminate abuse liability of the combination product. Euphoria is attenuated by naloxone, but some effect remains. Subjective response may vary depending on dosage; buprenorphine/naloxone 2 mg/0.5 mg has been compared to heroin or buprenorphine alone by drug abusers, whereas subjective effects of higher buprenorphine/naloxone doses were less favorable [7]. Nonetheless, a clear majority of drug users who frequently inject buprenorphine/naloxone rate the effect as "bad" compared to buprenorphine without naloxone. Approximately 20% of users report a similar experience whether injecting buprenorphine or buprenorphine/naloxone formulations [287].

The majority of heroin users inject buprenorphine for therapeutic purposes, including self-treatment of addiction (up to 56% to 97% of users) or prevention of withdrawal (5% to 90%) [287-290]. Lack of access to a treatment program, due to geographic or economic barriers, may also increase illicit use of buprenorphine [289]. In the U.S., approximately three quarters of intravenous drug abusers and half of non-intravenous abusers obtain and use buprenorphine illicitly because they cannot afford formal treatment [291]. Patients already enrolled in opioid dependence treatment may use additional buprenorphine illicitly because of insufficient dosing [3]. At other times, buprenorphine may serve as a substitute when an abuser's medication is scarce or more expensive.

While heroin remained fairly cheap and readily accessible in the U.S., its production and availability declined sharply worldwide between 2000 and 2001, particularly in European and Asian countries [292]. Investigators in these countries have reported that lack of access to heroin drove abuse of other drugs during the last decade, with the European Monitoring Centre for Drugs and Drug Addiction (EMCDDA) attesting that heroin abuse has largely been replaced by synthetic drugs such as fentanyl and buprenorphine [278, 293-294]. In addition to lower cost and more availability, buprenorphine has the advantage of higher purity [295-297]. When injected, the increased bioavailability of even small sublingual doses can produce a profound effect, and 29% of users select buprenorphine over heroin to save money [3, 294]. Some may elect to use buprenorphine due to the perception that they would be subject to less legal recourse and policing than if they were using heroin [3, 293]. A much smaller subset of abusers, usually 8% to 11% in surveys, inject buprenorphine for euphoria [287-289]. Some investigators have noted that more non-injectors use buprenorphine for this reason (69%) compared to IV drug users (32%) [291]. Less than 5% use buprenorphine to enhance the effects of other drugs [287-288]. Curiously, a significant number of users ingest buprenorphine for other therapeutic reasons, including 40% to 42% for treatment of psychiatric symptoms including anxiety or depression, and 47% to reduce pain [289]. Buprenorphine has been reported in at least one case of drug-facilitated sexual assault [298].

Prevalence

At first, buprenorphine was believed to have low abuse potential, and it could be obtained without restriction in some countries [295]. The first report of abuse originated in New Zealand in 1983, and several more followed [295, 299-300]. As medical professionals and legal authorities began to recognize the abuse liability of buprenorphine, several countries reclassified it as a prescription-only product and imposed restrictions on its use [3, 235, 295]. Clinicians began prescribing buprenorphine/naloxone once it was available, as it was less desirable to abusers than buprenorphine alone [7, 301]. In countries where the buprenorphine mono-product was available for some time prior to introduction of the combination buprenorphine/naloxone product, the prevalence of abuse became significant. In Finland, buprenorphine was introduced in 1981, and was legalized for the treatment of opioid withdrawal and maintenance in 2000. Buprenorphine/naloxone was introduced in 2004. Use has not been imposed with as many restrictions as the U.S., and under certain conditions buprenorphine can be dispensed by pharmacies [142]. By 2007, buprenorphine had overtaken heroin to become the primary drug of abuse. In surveys of intravenous abusers in Finnish maintenance programs, 73% identified buprenorphine as their most frequently abused drug, with 82% injecting at least once a day (most frequently 3 to 4 times per day) [287]. Similarly, 89% of heroin users in Sweden reported using buprenorphine during past year [288], and in India and Singapore, approximately half of intravenous drug users either began injecting with buprenorphine or reported buprenorphine as their primary drug of choice [293, 302-303]. Buprenorphine is the one of the most commonly injected drugs in India, second only to heroin [303].

Social, political, and economic factors may all influence abuse rates. In the U.S., the sublingual buprenorphine mono-product was never widely used due to the simultaneous approval of buprenorphine/naloxone. In addition, access to heroin was not limited as it was in European countries. These circumstances may have spared—or at least, delayed—widespread abuse of buprenorphine in the U.S. [3]. The first reported American cases of abuse and diversion occurred in Vermont in December 2005. Shortly thereafter, the SAMHSA CSAT commissioned a study of abuse and diversion of buprenorphine only to discover that both had increased since the approval of the sublingual products [63]. Still, buprenorphine was reported as the last primary drug of choice among patients enrolled in methadone maintenance treatment, relative to heroin and prescription opioids [63, 257]. Buprenorphine abuse and diversion increased from 2005 to 2009, though not as much as methadone, heroin, and oxycodone [279]. Following 2010, buprenorphine abuse increased more rapidly, coinciding with introduction of an abuse-deterrent oxycodone controlled-release formulation. Increases in abuse were also noted with oxymorphone, indicating that some patients may have switched their drug of choice in the aftermath of the oxycodone reformulation to a less abuse-deterrent form [304].

Reported trends for buprenorphine misuse in recent years reflect the significant increase in prescribing. ED visits related to buprenorphine climbed from 3,161 in 2005 to 34,863 in 2011, with approximately half due to nonmedical use [276, 305]. Hydrocodone and oxycodone are the most prevalent abused drugs in the U.S.; however, when corrected for the quantity of dosage units distributed to retail outlets, buprenorphine is ranked second among the opioids for nonmedical use resulting in ED visits [249, 306]. Buprenorphine is widely available in prison systems, and has been increasingly detected in biological specimens submitted from prison inmates and parolees [307]. More than half of states in the U.S. had one or more media reports of buprenorphine misuse or diversion in the first two thirds of 2012, with many reports coming from small urban, suburban, and rural areas with disproportionate levels of opioid abuse [249, 308].

Diversion

Buprenorphine is readily available on the black market worldwide [146, 307, 309]. The National Forensic Laboratory Information System (NFLIS), a Drug Enforcement Administration (DEA) program which collects information regarding drugs seized by law enforcement in the U.S., reported 446 seizures of buprenorphine in 2005 [279]. NFLIS reports of buprenorphine seizures continued, with highest prevalence in the Northeastern U.S. and 11,801 seizures reported nationwide in 2012. According to the latest reports, buprenorphine seizures rank 3rd among opioid analgesics: behind oxycodone and hydrocodone, but above morphine, methadone, and hydromorphone [310]. The primary source of diverted buprenorphine in the U.S. comes from physician-written prescriptions for the treatment of opioid dependence [63]. Reports of doctor shopping and medication borrowing for pill counts are increasingly common for buprenorphine in addition to other prescription opioids [63, 311]. Patients may divert sublingual doses, which has been a noted problem in Australian pharmacies where diversion may impact 22% to 33% of clients [312-313]. Other methods of diversion have been described, including theft and illegal importation [63]. Some reports have surfaced that buprenorphine cannot be detected by sniffer dogs, which may help smugglers to evade border drug control procedures [314].

Nearly half of intravenous buprenorphine users in an Australian study obtained medication illicitly, as do most out-of-treatment abusers in the U.S. and abroad [288, 291, 315]. Inconsistent accounts of diversion rates for specific formulations have arisen. Buprenorphine/naloxone is less subject to diversion with lower street values than the buprenorphine mono-products [101, 266, 287, 316]. In Finland, buprenorphine alone commands double the street price of buprenorphine/naloxone, but substantially less than heroin or amphetamine [287]. The margin is narrower in the U.S., with RADARS reporting a 17% price increase for buprenorphine versus abuse-deterrent formulations such as buprenorphine/naloxone [316]. Conversely, all formulations of buprenorphine had the same median street value in Australia [290]. If diversion is suspected, less than daily dosing under observed conditions can be performed [101].

Abuse Patterns

Abuse of buprenorphine more commonly occurs in opioid-experienced abusers [295-297]. Previous reported abuse of other drugs, especially tobacco and cannabis, may increase the likelihood of initiation of buprenorphine abuse [317]. Compared to amphetamine abusers in Finland, buprenorphine is associated with daily abuse with no drug-free months for the past year, and is more commonly observed in younger patients without psychotic symptoms [318]. Intravenous abuse of buprenorphine is more likely if patients are maintained on a low sublingual dose [7].

Injecting drug users who replace the buprenorphine mono-product with buprenorphine/naloxone typically increase the dose [319]. The tradeoff may be increased withdrawal symptoms secondary to the presence of naloxone; abusers may compensate for this effect and facilitate euphoria by abusing concomitant medications, particularly benzodiazepines or heroin [319-320]. Subjects who use buprenorphine with benzodiazepines or neuroleptics report that the combination affords a high similar to heroin abuse [146]. As a pattern of drug use, concomitant medications are a common modality for buprenorphine abuse. DAWN data indicates buprenorphine alone is involved in only 41% of ED visits related to nonmedical use [276]. Rates of polysubstance abuse have been reported between 72-100% in buprenorphine abusers [287, 293, 315].

Of all medications abused concomitantly with buprenorphine, benzodiazepine use is chiefly described and selected by 7-67% buprenorphine users [151, 287, 320]. Ingestion of benzodiazepines occurs in 27% of nonmedical buprenorphine-related ED visits [276]. In the U.S., alprazolam is the most frequently identified benzodiazepine ingested with buprenorphine [151]. In a large study of buprenorphine-positive urine specimens (>20,000) submitted for drug testing in the U.S., benzodiazepines were the most common non-prescribed medications detected with non-prescribed buprenorphine, detected in 34% specimens. Interestingly, benzodiazepines were also the most commonly prescribed drug in 21% of patients prescribed buprenorphine, more than all other prescription drugs combined [153]. The safety implication of the rate of benzodiazepine use in this population, either prescribed or illicit, is concerning.

Opioids are also abused concurrently with buprenorphine. DAWN data indicates opioid pain relievers are implicated in 12% of ED visits for nonmedical buprenorphine use [276]. According to buprenorphine-positive UDT results, oxycodone and hydrocodone were the next most prevalent non-prescribed drugs after benzodiazepines. These findings were significantly more common when buprenorphine was not prescribed (approximately 18% for oxycodone and 22% for hydrocodone), versus patients who were prescribed buprenorphine (13% positive for oxycodone, 11% positive for hydrocodone) [153]. Use of illicit drugs has also been described in 27% of nonmedical buprenorphine-related ED visits [276]. Rates of illicit drug use as detected by UDT for all users of buprenorphine in pain clinics ranged between 34% to 38%; these rates are much higher than the overall prevalence of illicit drugs in the pain population, which has been reported at 11% [153, 321].

Route

Buprenorphine may be abused by numerous routes, with injection identified as a common abuse method [39]. Sublingual tablets are water-soluble and easily crushed for intravenous abuse, though the dissolution process can take 3 to 8 minutes [48, 66]. Buprenorphine/naloxone is less appealing to injecting abusers, but is still commonly injected with one-third of subjects reporting withdrawal symptoms [31]. Among abusers who are regularly injecting, use of buprenorphine/naloxone is lower compared to buprenorphine alone, but comparable to methadone [313]. In Finland, 68% of intravenous drug abusers reported injecting buprenorphine/naloxone. Only 45% reported injecting buprenorphine/naloxone more than once, which suggests experimentation; only 8% reported frequent abuse [287]. Intravenous buprenorphine is less prevalent among Australian intravenous abusers, with rates between 32% and 37% [294, 315]. Only 10% listed buprenorphine as their preferred drug for injection [294]. When patients enrolled in buprenorphine treatment programs are surveyed, intravenous buprenorphine abuse is reported by 20% to 27% of patients in France and Australia, compared to 66% of methadone-maintained patients who inject methadone [211, 322].

Buprenorphine use is sometimes associated with less risky behaviors and a lower incidence of HIV [293, 323]. Compared to heroin users, intravenous buprenorphine abusers in India inject less frequently, have fewer people in their drug-using network, face fewer threats of arrest, and are less likely to share injection equipment. Nevertheless, it is worth noting that more than half of buprenorphine injectors in India and other countries admit to needle sharing [293, 318]. Other high risk behaviors that have been described among those injecting buprenorphine include unsafe needle disposal, inappropriate cleaning of needles, and unsafe sexual practices [303]. Needle sharing may increase risk of disease transmission, and intravenous buprenorphine use has been associated with infections such as abscesses, emboli, acute limb ischemia, endocarditis, sepsis, HIV, and hepatitis C [3, 211, 302, 319]. In treatment programs where sublingual dosing is supervised, diversion can increase the risk of infection because microbial flora present from patient's mouth may remain on the tablets [3, 294]. The majority of injected doses are dispensed under unsupervised conditions [290].

Snorting has also been reported as a common route of buprenorphine abuse. Intranasal administration results in more rapid effects than sublingual use, with onset occurring as rapidly as 10 minutes [2, 31, 35, 39] Naloxone demonstrates increased bioavailability via the intranasal versus sublingual route; however, intranasal administration of both buprenorphine and buprenorphine/naloxone produce increases in subjective and physiologic mu receptor effects [39-42]. In one study of intranasal administration, abusers reported higher subjective ratings and street value for buprenorphine 8 mg compared to buprenorphine/naloxone 8 mg/2 mg, but this difference was not statistically significant [39]. In addition to snorting, smoking has appeared in some reports as the most common intranasal administration method [314, 324-325].

Among patients enrolled in opioid maintenance in Australia, 18% reported having inhaled buprenorphine or buprenorphine/naloxone. Recent inhalation was rare, and most patients used this route as experimentation rather than a preferred mode of use [325].

Abuse of transdermal buprenorphine increases the risk for overdose and death [8]. Transdermal administration produces less intense and delayed opioid effects and relatively low plasma concentrations, thus lending a potentially lower abuse potential than parenteral buprenorphine; yet, patients may abuse patches by chewing or extracting buprenorphine for parenteral use [2, 326]. The buprenorphine/naloxone film is also subject to intravenous abuse, with a frequency of injection similar to methadone and buprenorphine/naloxone sublingual tablets [290]. Overall, it appears intravenous administration is a preferred route by buprenorphine abusers, with prevalence of 43% to 60%. Abuse by snorting or smoking has been reported in 5% to 29% of abusers. Sublingual abuse has been reported with varying prevalence, as low as 14% in some studies, or as the most common route of administration in others [287-288].

Practitioners must be vigilant when prescribing buprenorphine, as abuse of concomitant medications and intravenous abuse can result in very poor outcomes for patients. Burgeoning rates of buprenorphine abuse may be of concern to physicians not prescribing buprenorphine as well, particularly those practicing in pain management, as patients abusing other opioids may select buprenorphine if their drug of choice is not available. However, illicit use of buprenorphine may be associated with positive aspects. Buprenorphine users may experience reduced risk for harm compared to other opioids or injectable drugs, with lower rates of mortality and lower high-risk behaviors [3].

FATAL OVERDOSES

Escalations in buprenorphine prescribing patterns and increased availability have been associated with overdoses and fatalities. From 2002 to 2011, the Utah Poison Control Center reported a 13-fold increase in buprenorphine exposures [277]. The American Association of Poison Control Centers reported 3,625 cases and three deaths involving buprenorphine in 2011 [5]. Deaths associated with buprenorphine have repeatedly been reported in literature, particularly from countries where buprenorphine is extensively used [59, 86, 135, 142, 144-147, 298, 309]. In a study of more than 1300 postmortem cases in Finland, buprenorphine was found in 29% of opioid-positive cases [142]. It is difficult to assess true prevalence of drug-related deaths, and cases associated with buprenorphine may be underestimated [309, 327]. In previous years, laboratories did not have suitable analytical capabilities to detect buprenorphine or norbuprenorphine [309, 328].

Buprenorphine-related cases may not be properly identified if medical examiners do not specifically request buprenorphine analysis [63].

Several risk factors are recurrently linked with buprenorphine fatalities and include co-ingestion of psychotropic drugs (e.g., benzodiazepines), availability of high-dose formulations, and intravenous administration of crushed tablets [144, 309]. Respiratory depression requiring mechanical ventilation has been associated with intravenous administration of 2-10 mcg/kg. To put this in perspective, an 8 mg tablet of buprenorphine provides 10-50 times this dose [144]. The combination of buprenorphine and naloxone may not decrease risk for overdose death in comparison to buprenorphine alone. An evaluation of 225 buprenorphine-related deaths identified buprenorphine/naloxone in the majority of cases, and twice as often as buprenorphine alone. In one study, parenteral buprenorphine/naloxone was presumed to be involved in 12.4% of the cases based upon urine concentrations [329]. Sole ingestion of buprenorphine has rarely been associated with fatal overdose, but cases have been described that indicate respiratory depression can still occur [59, 142]. According to a study by Seldén *et al.*, buprenorphine was the only drug identified in 10% of postmortem cases [59].

Polydrug use in postmortem cases is very common [330]. Benzodiazepines are frequently co-ingested and this drug-drug interaction does not appear to be dose-dependent [59, 135, 142, 144-147, 298, 309]. Alprazolam has been found to be involved in 40% of death cases and hypnotics/sedatives in 75% [59]. Other neuroleptics such as antidepressants and antipsychotics have also been detected [309]. Alcohol use may be a risk factor and has been frequently detected in conjunction with buprenorphine in overdose cases, with reported rates as high as 58% of postmortem cases [142, 324, 330]. An additional component that may increase susceptibility for fatal overdose is reduced drug tolerance due to a period of abstinence [330-333]. Tolerance may be reduced over a period of time as short as a few days up to a period of weeks [330]. Hair analysis has been used to demonstrate abstinence in weeks or months leading up to heroin overdose [333]. Even so, concomitant drug ingestion may play a more significant role in overdose deaths, as subjects with opioid-negative hair samples (suggesting reduced tolerance) have been found to have similar blood morphine concentrations to opioid-dependent subjects in heroin fatalities, and additional drugs were often present [330].

Experts agree that buprenorphine concentration data alone often does not clearly point to cause of death. Differences in concentrations between postmortem cases attributed to buprenorphine and those attributed to other causes have not been shown to be clinically significant [142]. Notably, buprenorphine concentrations are often found within a therapeutic range [135, 142, 144-147, 298, 309, 327]. Reported concentration data for buprenorphine and norbuprenorphine in postmortem cases are presented in Table 2. Benzodiazepine concentrations in postmortem cases are also often found at therapeutic concentrations as well [59, 142, 147, 298]. Given these findings, a specific lethal concentration cannot be defined for buprenorphine, particularly in the presence of other drugs [59]. Postmortem blood concentrations of buprenorphine are often less than 30 ng/mL [2]. Low blood concentrations may suggest delayed onset of respiratory depression [59, 330]. Buprenorphine-related deaths may occur immediately post-exposure, as demonstrated in 10% of cases in one study; however, time to death is often delayed and death during sleep has been reported in up to 50% of cases [59, 142].

The median ratio of buprenorphine/norbuprenorphine in blood has been found to be 1.8 in buprenorphine poisoning cases, compared to a median ratio of 0.86 for other causes of death. Consequently, a ratio greater than one may be suggestive of acute overdose [142]. Low concentrations of norbuprenorphine in urine are suggestive of drug abstinence or acute overdose, as buprenorphine/ norbuprenorphine ratios may be >1 for the first 7 hours post-dose [334].

When considering mortality related to drug abuse, overall trends must be considered. Unfortunately, decreases in deaths associated with one drug are often accompanied by increases in deaths attributed to another. While buprenorphine-related fatalities have accompanied increasing use of the drug, mortality related to other drugs of abuse has decreased significantly according to several reports. In Finland, an increase in buprenorphine abuse and mortality was accompanied by a noticeable decline in heroin deaths from 2000 and 2004 [287]. In France, a five-fold decrease in deaths attributable to heroin was observed between 1995 and 2003 [235]. In proportion to prescribing rates, buprenorphine deaths are estimated to be three-fold lower than deaths due to methadone in France, where buprenorphine is widely prescribed and abused [3, 327]. Similarly, in Germany the proportion of deaths involving methadone far outnumbered the one reported death involving buprenorphine.

In the geographical region of the study, only an estimated 10% of those involved in opioid treatment received buprenorphine as the treatment intervention and heroin was detected in more than 60% of cases.

However, the rate of deaths with methadone was proportionally higher than buprenorphine [335]. These trends undoubtedly occur as a result of buprenorphine's improved safety profile.

Table 2. Postmortem concentrations of buprenorphine and norbuprenorphine in biological specimens

Specimen Type	Concentrations (ng/mL)	BUP/NBUP Ratio	Cases	Method	LOQ	Ref.
Blood	BUP (hydrolysis unknown): 1.1 – 29; mean 8.4 NBUP (hydrolysis unknown): 0.2 – 12.6; mean 2.6	Mean 8.5 (0.5 – 36)	20 fatalities	HPLC/ MS	BUP: 0.1 ng/mL NBUP: 0.2 ng/mL	144
Blood	Total BUP: 3,276 Total NBUP: 399	8.2	1 fatality	LC-ES-ES	Not provided	148
Blood	BUP (hydrolysis unknown): 0.1 – 76 NBUP (hydrolysis unknown): <0.1 – 65	0.5 – 2.5 for 5 typical cases	117 fatalities	HPLC/ MS or GC/MS	BUP 0.2 ng/mL NBUP 0.1 ng/mL	309
Blood	BUP (hydrolysis unknown): 0.3 – 7.7; mean 3.5 NBUP (hydrolysis unknown): 0.3-16.2, mean 2.9	Mean 2.2 (0.4 – 6.8)	13 fatalities	HPLC/ MS	BUP 0.2 ng/mL NBUP 0.1 ng/mL	146
Blood	BUP (hydrolysis unknown): 0 – 68.6 NBUP (hydrolysis unknown): 0 – 26.9	– 5.0 For 4 cases	21 fatalities	LC/MS	BUP 0.25 ng/mL NBUP 1.25 ng/mL	147
Blood	Total BUP: 7.1 – 15.4; Free BUP: 3.8 – 6.2 Total NBUP: 2.8 – 4.5; Free NBUP: 0.56 – 1.5	3.3 – 6.8 (free) 1.3 – 5.5 (total)	3 fatalities	HPLC/ MS/MS	Not provided	324
Femoral Blood	BUP + NBUP (hydrolysis unknown): 1.1 – 17.7; mean 7.4; median 5.8	n/a	6 fatalities	HPLC/ MS	Not provided	145
Femoral Blood	BUP (hydrolysis unknown): 1.1 NBUP (hydrolysis unknown): 0.2	5.5	1 fatality (child)	HPLC-MS	BUP 0.2 ng/mL NBUP 0.1 ng/mL	298

Table 2. (Continued)

Specimen Type	Concentrations (ng/mL)	BUP/NBUP Ratio	Cases	Method	LOQ	Ref.
Femoral Blood	BUP (hydrolysis unknown): 0.002 – 100 NBUP (hydrolysis unknown): 0.14 – 200	Median 1.8 Median 0.86	182 BUP poisoning 209 other	LC/MS/MS and GC/MS	0.2 ng/mL	329
Whole Blood	BUP (hydrolysis unknown): 0.5 – 46.1	n/a	34 fatalities	GC/MS	1 ng/mL	135
Pooled Blood	Free BUP: 52 Free NBUP: 39	1.3	1 fatality (child)	LC/MS/MS	Not provided	132
Urine	Total BUP: 4 – 1,033 Total NBUP: 6.6 – 230	Mean 2.7 (0.4 – 8.3)	20 fatalities	HPLC/MS	BUP: 0.1 ng/mL NBUP: 0.2 ng/mL	144
Urine	BUP (hydrolysis unknown): 15 – 344.1; mean 69	n/a	6 fatalities	HPLC/MS	Not provided	145
Urine	Total BUP: 3,397 Total NBUP: 624	5.4	1 fatality	LC-ES-MS	Not provided	148
Urine	Free BUP: 9.1 Free NBUP: 9.6	0.95	1 fatality (child)	HPLC-MS	BUP: 0.2 ng/mL NBUP: 0.1 ng/mL	298
Urine	BUP (hydrolysis unknown): 0 – 33.8	n/a	9 fatalities	GC/MS	1 ng/mL	135
Urine	BUP (hydrolysis unknown): 0 – 73.6 NBUP (hydrolysis unknown): 0 – 359	Mean 0.9 (0.2 – 2.9)	21 fatalities	LC/MS/MS	BUP 0.5 ng/mL NBUP 2.5 ng/mL	147
Urine	Total BUP: 193 – 775; Free BUP: 21 – 43.5 Total NBUP: 22 –39; Free NBUP: 6 – 17	1.3 – 3.5 (free) 4.9 – 9.8 (total)	3 fatalities	HPLC/MS/MS	Not provided	324

* Buprenorphine (BUP), norbuprenorphine (NBUP).

On the whole, the benefits of buprenorphine availability may outweigh harm, but healthcare providers and patients should be aware that misuse of buprenorphine is not without risk.

Compliance Monitoring

Patient compliance with prescribed medications may be assessed through multiple methods including pill counts, substance abuse risk assessment tools (in cases where buprenorphine is used for pain management), prescription monitoring programs, and toxicological analysis [3]. International guidelines recommend use of an objective method to evaluate compliance, and UDT is the most commonly used assessment of this kind [94, 336]. In addition to evaluating patient compliance with prescribed medications, use of other drugs (e.g., benzodiazepines, alcohol, barbiturates, illicit drugs) can interfere with intended treatment and should be objectively assessed through toxicology testing at least monthly [94]. For patients receiving buprenorphine maintenance treatment, a thrice weekly schedule serves to maximize detection of illicit use and avoid repeatedly identifying single use for most medications, which could occur with daily analysis [337].

Studies of urine specimens from patients prescribed buprenorphine indicate compliance (buprenorphine positive result) in 83 – 90% of patients [153, 338]. Due to the prevalence of misuse/abuse as previously described, buprenorphine may often be an unexpected finding in toxicology results for clinical cases. Melanson *et al.* found 3.2% of chronic pain patients were unexpectedly positive for buprenorphine by random UDT [339]. In another study, the most prevalent medications detected in more than 300,000 urine specimens from pain management patients were (in order): hydrocodone, oxycodone, benzodiazepines, gabapentin, and buprenorphine. Buprenorphine had a similar positivity rate to morphine [340].

Toxicology Methods

Toxicological analysis of buprenorphine and its relevant markers can present analytical challenges. Several different methods for buprenorphine analysis have been described: gas chromatography-electron capture detection (GC-ECD), radioimmunoassay, liquid chromatography-electron capture detection (LC-ECD), gas chromatography/mass spectrometry (GC/MS), and liquid chromatography/tandem mass spectrometry (LC/MS/MS) [47, 328, 341-352]. The most common methods employed are immunoassay, GC/MS, and LC/MS/MS.

Immunoassay (IA)

IA is a common screening method for drugs of abuse or compliance testing. It uses the principle of competitive binding with a drug of interest, a labeled target, and an antibody. If a drug is present, it displaces a labeled target from binding to the antibody, yielding a presumptive positive result. IA tests may be sensitive but are not specific, as antibodies may bind to other structurally similar compounds. The sensitivity of an antibody to varying compounds is termed cross-reactivity, and high cross-reactivity with unrelated drugs may yield false positives [353].

Buprenorphine does not usually react to opiate IA tests, and a targeted IA test for buprenorphine is necessary [354-356]. Buprenorphine IA tests are widely available and are used at the point-of-care and in reference laboratories. Cross-reactivity with specific buprenorphine analytes may vary from assay to assay.

In some cases, cross-reactivity to norbuprenorphine may be less than 1%, and cross-reactivity to glucuronides may be low for some assays but acceptable for others [357-362]. Assays with high cross-reactivity to buprenorphine and norbuprenorphine but low detection of glucuronide conjugates have also been described [362-363].

Although buprenorphine assays are usually designed not to cross-react with other opiates, there have been some noted exceptions, illustrating the importance of confirming presumptive results by more specific methods. Immunalysis' ELISA targeted to buprenorphine did not cross-react with 10 ng/mL of dihydrocodeine, codeine, tramadol, morphine, methadone, or EDDP (methadone metabolite) [361]. However, various medications have been associated with false positives upon testing by cloned enzyme donor immunoassay (CEDIA) buprenorphine assays and are listed below:

- Tramadol [359]
- Dihydrocodeine [200]
- Morphine, codeine, and methadone [364]

- Chloroquine and hydroxychloroquine [357]
- Morphine, codeine, dihydrocodeine; amisulpride or sulpiride [365]

As evidenced by variability in cross-reactivity and the potential for false positives and false negatives, IA methods have limitations when used in clinical and forensic applications. A study examining an automatic on-site test and a fluorescence polarization immunoassay (FPIA)-based device concluded more sensitive instrumentation was needed for the workplace setting, as 0% sensitivities were found for concentrations up to twice the thresholds [366]. Although Abbott's FPIA product is no longer available, some IA tests may have similar performance. Use of the CEDIA reagent for buprenorphine yielded false negative results, failing to identify recent intake even shortly after single-dose ingestion [334]. IA tests may frequently exhibit low sensitivities to the most abundantly excreted metabolites, which can be a significant limitation when IA is used to monitor compliance [357-362].

Several comparison studies of IA have been made to mass spectrometry (MS) methods such as GC/MS [200, 358, 360-361, 363, 367]. The buprenorphine LUCIO Nal Von Minden assay (on a Roche COBAS Integra 800 analyzer) was compared to GC/MS for workplace testing. Investigators concluded a 5 ng/mL threshold provided acceptable sensitivity and specificity for buprenorphine screening in the workplace setting with 100% sensitivity, 88% specificity, and an overall agreement of 94% [362]. In contrast, a 10 ng/mL threshold resulted in 90% sensitivity, 100% specificity, and an overall agreement of 94%, leading the investigators to conclude the 5 ng/mL threshold may be more appropriate for workplace testing. Hull *et al.* compared the Microgenics CEDIA buprenorphine assay to LC/MS/MS analysis and determined that a 5 ng/mL buprenorphine threshold led to 97.9% agreement in results. In the same study, a 20 ng/mL threshold resulted in false negatives with a 61.5% negative predictive value. The CEDIA assay demonstrated comparable cross-reactivity to buprenorphine and buprenorphine-glucuronide and negligible (< 0.015%) cross-reactivity to norbuprenorphine and norbuprenorphine-glucuronide [367]. Consequently, presumptive positives identified by the assay may indicate more recent or consistent buprenorphine ingestion.

The influence of drug-drug interactions on parent drug/metabolite ratios should not be underestimated, and true compliance may be overlooked when some IA methods are applied. More sensitive and specific methods such as

MS-based tests offer advantages in detection of relevant metabolites compared to immunoassay technology.

Mass Spectrometry (MS)

MS-based methods offer greater sensitivity and specificity and can be targeted to both buprenorphine and norbuprenorphine. Mass spectrometry analyses also allow for an extended period of detection relative to IA methods, although this varies depending upon which analytes are included in the method and what thresholds are in use.

Generally confirmations are performed following presumptive positive results by IA; however, some paradigms utilize direct testing by MS methods to reduce the risk of false negatives [356]. The true impact of false negatives in certain populations should not be underestimated and index MS testing should be strongly considered if a false negative will significantly impact clinical care. Testing directly by MS can also assist in interpretation by providing quantitative data for parent drug and/or metabolites. Many laboratories have utilized LC/MS/MS for analysis of buprenorphine [352, 367-370].

LC/MS/MS methods may offer superior sensitivity compared to GC/MS, enabling use of lower thresholds [371]. GC/MS analysis also requires additional process steps including extractions and derivatization that may increase required sample volume and testing time over LC/MS/MS analysis [47, 349-350].

Analysis of buprenorphine presents certain analytical and interpretive challenges. Buprenorphine has unfavorable fragmentation in the ion source which may compromise sensitivity, particularly when it is included in methods with other drugs.

Analyses must also be capable of detecting a wide range of concentrations, especially in urine and oral fluid. Potential for carryover (which can result in false positive tests) should be assessed carefully when mass spectrometry methods are used for buprenorphine in clinical testing; otherwise, contamination false positives may occur for neighboring samples of highly positive specimens [372].

Carryover risk may vary depending on the analyte, extraction procedures, and the method; one investigation found lower risk with LC/MS/MS versus GC/MS (though the same level of risk may not hold true for all GC/MS and LC/MS/MS methods) [349]. Adulteration attempts through addition of drug directly to urine post-collection or recent sublingual administration preceding oral fluid collection can lead to very high concentrations and increase risk for laboratory contamination error unless appropriate quality control measures are in place [373].

Blood/Plasma

Blood or plasma monitoring of buprenorphine may be performed, though it is rarely done in routine clinical testing. Peak plasma concentrations of buprenorphine and norbuprenorphine are generally comparable and fairly low relative to most opioids [48, 374]. Therapeutic concentrations of buprenorphine typically range from 2 ng/mL to 20 ng/mL [146]. It has been suggested that plasma levels > 0.7 ng/mL are required to suppress withdrawal symptoms [183]. Blood buprenorphine levels have rarely exceeded 10 ng/mL in most studies, and the exceptions are generally observed with higher doses (i.e., 32 mg/day) [26, 29, 31, 33, 46]. A large amount of intra-individual and inter-individual variability exists, but concentrations tend to increase with increasing doses [84, 375]. Moderate correlations have been observed between trough levels and dosage strength of buprenorphine tablets, but not with dosage strength of the film [66]. The period of detection is highly variable, ranging from 7 hours following sublingual administration using a threshold of 0.2 ng/mL, up to 24 to 96 hours at a threshold of 0.1 ng/mL [48, 371]. Plasma norbuprenorphine concentrations normally exceed those of buprenorphine with chronic dosing [45, 183] or when specimens are collected further out from time of ingestion. An average pre-dose plasma ratio of norbuprenorphine/buprenorphine of 3 may be observed during chronic dosing [34].

Peak concentrations for low doses of sublingual buprenorphine may fall below ng/mL thresholds. Maximum concentrations (Cmax) in plasma following 4 mg SL administration ranged from 0.81 – 7.2 ng/mL; in other studies, subnanogram concentrations of buprenorphine have been noted within 24 hours following SL administration [26, 371]. Single-dose administration of buprenorphine/naloxone 8/2 mg SL resulted in a Cmax range of 2.2 – 2.8 ng/mL and 1.5 – 2.4 ng/mL for buprenorphine and norbuprenorphine, respectively [48]. Mean steady state plasma concentration during days 21 – 35 of chronic administration of 8 mg SL daily was 0.8 ng/mL for buprenorphine and 1.1 ng/mL for norbuprenorphine [376]. In substitution treatment patients receiving SL doses of 1 – 16 mg/day, mean serum concentrations ranged from

1.1 – 8.5 ng/mL by semi-quantitative methods [377]. Norbuprenorphine may peak 0.5 to 1.5 hours later than buprenorphine in plasma following single-dose administration [34, 48, 374].

Transdermal use of buprenorphine typically produces subnanogram[a]/mL concentrations of buprenorphine. Consequently, much more sensitive assays are required for measurements. Plasma AUC values are dose-proportional and did not change over a 60-day period. After a single-dose application, Cmax steady state concentrations for 5 mcg/hour, 10 mcg/hour, and 20 mcg/hour ranged from 176 – 471 pg/mL and after repeated applications, Cmax concentration for 10 mcg/h was 224 pg/mL [8]. Examinations of buprenorphine concentrations and patient age have shown similar concentrations in patients aged 50 – 60 years old and patients aged ≥ 75 years old who received two doses of transdermal buprenorphine 5 mcg/h every 7 days. Overall, buprenorphine concentrations ranged from 13 – 169 pg/mL and norbuprenorphine concentrations ranged from ranged 13 – 57 pg/mL. Mean Cmax steady state concentration of buprenorphine was 83 pg/mL in patients aged 50 – 60 years and 72 pg/mL in those ≥ 75 years. The mean Cmax steady state concentration for norbuprenorphine was 22 pg/mL for patients aged 50 – 60 years and 20 pg/mL in those ≥ 75 years. The mean minimum concentration (Cmin) at steady state was 47 pg/mL in both groups. Norbuprenorphine ranged from 13 – 57 pg/mL, with a mean Cmin steady state concentration of 14 pg/mL and 16 pg/mL in the younger and older groups, respectively [111].

Following implantation of subdermal buprenorphine, mean buprenorphine Cmax ranged from 2 – 3 ng/mL and time to maximum concentration (Tmax) averaged 16 – 17 h. Tmax for norbuprenorphine was 6 hours post insertion, which was attributed to sublingual buprenorphine use prior to implantation. Time to steady state was estimated to be approximately 21 days and the average buprenorphine concentrations during this phase were 0.4 – 0.7 ng/mL. Norbuprenorphine concentrations averaged 0.12 – 0.32 ng/mL over the six month period [378].

Increased clearance during pregnancy may alter buprenorphine plasma concentrations, depending on trimester [116, 225]. In pregnant women receiving 1 – 28 mg/day of SL buprenorphine (median dose 8.5 mg/day), plasma concentrations were 0.6 – 1.4 ng/mL (mean 1 ng/mL) for buprenorphine and 0.9 – 1.4 ng/mL (mean 1.2 ng/mL) for norbuprenorphine [379]. Following 14 – 20 mg SL administration, plasma concentrations were 0 – 35.2 ng/mL (median 1.3 ng/mL) for buprenorphine, 0 – 27.5 ng/mL (median

[a] One nanogram (ng) is equal to 1,000 picgorams (pg)

2.9 ng/mL) for norbuprenorphine, 0 – 32.1 ng/mL (median 1.7 ng/mL) for buprenorphine-glucuronide, and 1.5 – 81.2 ng/mL (median 14.3 ng/mL) for norbuprenorphine-glucuronide [380]. One study compared mean trough levels between sublingual tablet and film formulations and found no differences. Concentrations ranged from 1.5 – 3.5 ng/mL after administration of 4 – 32 mg/day [66].

Naloxone may be detected following sublingual administration only when very low thresholds (0.025 – 0.5 ng/mL) are used. In subjects receiving chronic dosing of buprenorphine 16 mg/naloxone 4 mg SL, naloxone was detected for 2 hours post-dose in all cases, and for up to 4 hours in one subject. Naloxone Cmax was 0.139 ng/mL and Tmax was 0.5 h. Nornaloxone was not detected in any of the subjects. [56]. Higher concentrations may suggest injection or intranasal administration of buprenorphine/naloxone.

URINE

Urine drug testing is routinely performed as part of compliance assessment in pain management and opioid dependence treatment programs. Urinary buprenorphine concentrations are often 10 to 100-fold lower than those observed for other opioids, which can create challenges for measurement of buprenorphine in urine. While excretion patterns vary, overall trends have been reported in the literature. Urine largely contains the following analytes, in order from highest to lowest concentration: norbuprenorphine glucuronide, buprenorphine glucuronide, and norbuprenorphine. Many studies have detected very small quantities of parent compound [47, 49, 225, 341, 351, 381]. In a large study of chronic pain patients, the addition of norbuprenorphine to buprenorphine analysis performed by LC/MS/MS increased detection rate by 10% [368]. Due to extensive metabolism by UGT enzymes, free buprenorphine and free norbuprenorphine urine concentrations are low. Fox *et al.* established the proportion of free buprenorphine was 6.4% (range 0 – 67%) and free norbuprenorphine was 34% (range 0 – 100%) [349]. Accordingly, urine specimens are usually analyzed following hydrolysis, otherwise false negatives for buprenorphine may result [381-382].

Similar to laboratory analysis of morphine, hydrolysis of buprenorphine specimens may be performed by pre-treatment with beta-glucuronidase [352]. The increase in buprenorphine concentration after hydrolysis was approximately 50% with a radioimmunoassay method [342]. Norbuprenorphine-glucuronide is cleaved less efficiently than buprenorphine-glucuronide by glucuronidase [348, 352]. Factors such as source of enzyme, temperature, and incubation time may affect hydrolysis efficiency [267, 383]. Norbuprenorphine-3-glucuronide completely hydrolyzed by β-glucuronidase from E. *coli* or H. *pomatia* at 60°C for 4 hours [383]. On the other hand, acidic and basic hydrolysis processes were not shown to be satisfactory. For example, the hydrolysis process for buprenorphine-3-glucuronide was very slow and only 2% was hydrolyzed after 2 h at 50°C [267]. Hydrolysis processes may take longer for norbuprenorphine-3-glucuronide compared to buprenorphine-3-glucuronide. Therefore, the rate of hydrolysis may lead to false negatives with some methods, and is of clinical relevance when interpreting parent and metabolite ratios [383]. Ideally, laboratories should evaluate hydrolysis efficiency in their method validation.

Some analytical methods use direct measurement of glucuronide conjugates rather than employing a hydrolysis step [349, 352, 356, 384]. Al-Asmari *et al.* found higher total concentrations by means of direct measurement compared to β-glucuronidase hydrolysis, presumably due to incomplete hydrolysis [382]. However, direct analysis (referred to as "dilute-and-shoot" methods) without extraction may increase risk of ion suppression with electrospray LC/MS/MS, which may in turn chiefly affect glucuronide conjugates due to coelution and interference from other polar compounds or salts in urine. Solid phase extraction has been suggested to alleviate this effect, but it is worth noting that each analytical method will invariably demonstrate its own advantages and disadvantages [348, 384].

Due to variability of urine concentrations from changes in fluid intake or inter-patient differences in pharmacokinetic parameters, reliable correlations or buprenorphine or naloxone dose to resulting urine concentrations do not exist [222]. Concentrations frequently overlap in abusers and those using buprenorphine within established clinical parameters. In fact, total buprenorphine concentrations in abusers have been reported to be as low as 2.3 ng/mL, though lower values in abusers may be consistent with ingestion several days before specimen collection [348]. In opioid treatment patients, half of the urinary buprenorphine concentrations were < 100 ng/mL [200]. Unless otherwise specified, concentrations in this section represent total, post-hydrolysis concentrations.

Excretion patterns of parent drug and/or metabolite show significant inter-patient variability in the same manner as urinary drug concentrations. In 650 pain management patients, the majority of specimens (86.8%) were positive for both buprenorphine and norbuprenorphine, 4.2% were positive for buprenorphine-only, and 9.1% for norbuprenorphine-only. Total concentrations of norbuprenorphine-only results were significantly lower than overall norbuprenorphine distribution, with mean 129 ng/mL, median 9.6 ng/mL, and range 2.6 – 1,647 ng/mL. The presence of urinary norbuprenorphine in absence or parent drug is consistent with norbuprenorphine accumulation with chronic dosing [368]. A smaller study including 134 patients reported 78.4% positive for both buprenorphine and norbuprenorphine; norbuprenorphine-only was detected in 19.4% of specimens [370]. Norbuprenorphine-only results were again associated with lower concentrations, likely due to residual excretion [338]. Urine concentrations have been reported over a broad range of 0.5 – 979,000 ng/mL for buprenorphine and 1 – 25,000 ng/mL for norbuprenorphine, though concentrations <1,000 ng/mL are more common [84, 200, 222, 334, 340, 346, 348, 350-352, 358, 361, 367-368, 386-387]. Representative ranges from published studies are listed in Table 3.

Buprenorphine is not included in federally-regulated workplace testing by SAMHSA. The European Workplace Drug Testing Society (EWDTS) utilizes a 5 ng/mL threshold for both screening and confirmation, while Italy utilizes 10 ng/mL and 5 ng/mL thresholds for screening and confirmation, respectively. Positives for buprenorphine are ostensibly rare in Italy's workplace setting [385]. In clinical settings, particularly when buprenorphine compliance assessment is desired, false negatives are a heightened concern. A threshold of 1 ng/mL has been recommended for increased sensitivity in clinical patients; a higher 20 ng/mL threshold resulted in false negatives in 12% of abusers [348].

Norbuprenorphine/buprenorphine ratios are unrelated to dose in pain patients/addicts, and interpretation of ratios may be negatively biased by analytical methods if norbuprenorphine hydrolysis is incomplete [346, 348]. Studies indicate an overall range of norbuprenorphine/buprenorphine ratios between 0.067 – 27 with mean values reported between 2 – 4 [200, 222, 348, 361, 367, 382]. Ratios have trended lower in abuse cases, indicating higher concentrations of buprenorphine relative to norbuprenorphine [328, 361]. In eighteen volunteers who received 0.4 mg SL, norbuprenorphine/buprenorphine ratios > 1 were found at 7 hours post-dose. A ratio < 0.5 may indicate recent ingestion, and a ratio equal to 1 may suggest ingestion within the previous 7 to 10 hours [334]. A ratio of 3 has been demonstrated with ingestion 24 hours prior to urine collection, and may be noted before dosing during chronic treatment [59, 334,346]. Heikman *et al.* assessed total norbuprenorphine/ buprenorphine ratios in opioid-dependent subjects undergoing treatment: 90 – 94% had a ratio >1, particularly if samples were collected 24 hours after the last dose. Subjects in Group 0 (prior to maintenance treatment) had a mean ratio of 1.5, median ratio of 1.6, and a range of 0.5 – 2.6. In Group 1 (stable treatment phase), the mean ratio was 6.1, median 6.5, and the range 1 – 10. Group 2 subjects (unstable phase of treatment) had a mean ratio of 7.6, median 3.6, and a range of 0.4 – 27 [222].

Free norbuprenorphine/buprenorphine ratios were evaluated by McMillin *et al.,* with higher ratios reported than those observed with total norbuprenorphine and buprenorphine measurements.

Table 3. Urinary concentration data for buprenorphine and metabolites

Population	Method	LOQ	Concentrations (ng/mL)	Ref.
Opioid Maintenance	GC/MS	BUP 1.5 ng/mL NBUP 6 ng/mL	Total BUP: 0.5 – 2,936 Total NBUP: 4.0 – 4,462	200
ED, Maintenance, Autopsy	HPLC-ES-MS	1 ng/mL	Total BUP: 1.2 – 1,052 Total NBUP: Not provided	358
Pain Management	LC/MS/MS	BUP 1 ng/mL NBUP 2.5 ng/mL	Total BUP: 1 – 116,990; mean 381.2 +/- 208.9; median 48.8 Total NBUP: 2.6 – 3,026; mean 277.6 +/- 13.9; median 156.3	368
Detoxification	GC/MS	4 ng/mL	Total BUP: 28 – 1,458 Total NBUP: 27 – 1,843	346
Law, Prison, Probation, Hospital	LC/MS/MS	BUP-G 4.6 ng/mL NBUP-G 11.8 ng/mL	BUP-G: 6-161 NBUP-G: 12-295	350
Opioid Maintenance	LC/MS/MS	1 ng/mL	Total BUP: 8.9-2,000 Total NBUP: 14-2,700	222
Opioid Maintenance	LC-ESI/MS/MS	BUP, BUP-G, NBUP-G 0.5 ng/mL NBUP 2.5 ng/mL	Free BUP: 0.94 +/- 0.67 Free NBUP: 112 +/- 58 BUP-3-G: 94.9 +/- 27 NBUP-3-G: 662 +/- 219	351
Healthy Volunteers	LC/MS/MS	0.1 ng/mL	BUP (hydrolysis unknown): Cmax Range: 21.6-174.8 NBUP (hydrolysis unknown): Cmax Range: 1.2-6.8	84
Opioid Maintenance	LC/MS/MS	5 ng/mL	Total BUP: 0 – 1,200; mean 161 (SD 223); 15% less than 5 Total NBUP: 0 – 1,200	367
Healthy Volunteers	LC/MS/MS	0.5 ng/mL	Total BUP: peak 4.4 – 60 Total NBUP: peak 5.7 – 26	334
Detoxification and Probation	LC/MS/MS	Not provided	Total BUP: 2.9 – 1,080 Total NBUP: 5 – 2,580	348
Clinical	LC/MS/MS	BUP, NBUP 2 ng/mL	Free BUP: median 6.1; 9.8% higher than 1,000	352

Population	Method	LOQ	Concentrations (ng/mL)	Ref.
		BUP-G, NBUP-G 5 ng/mL	Free NBUP: median 64.7; few higher than 1,000 BUP-3-G: median 108 NBUP-3-G: 432	
Opioid Maintenance and Routine Lab Specimens	LC/MS/MS	1.3 ng/mL	Total BUP: 1 – 7,550 Total NBUP: 7 – 1,931	361
Pain Management	LC/MS/MS	10 ng/mL	Total BUP 97.5th percentile: 1,100 (nonparametric) Total NBUP 97.5th percentile: 3,894 (nonparametric)	386
Pain Management	LC/MS/MS	5 ng/mL	Total BUP 97th percentile: 1,296	387
Pain Management	LC/MS/MS	BUP 10 ng/mL NBUP 20 ng/mL	BUP (hydrolysis unknown): 10 – 979,135; mean 130.6; median 123.5 NBUP (hydrolysis unknown): 20 – 25,393; mean 343.2; median 370.0	340
Detoxification	GC/MS	BUP 0.25 ng/mL NBUP 0.20 ng/mL	Total BUP: 1,007 – 3,316 ng/mg creatinine Total NBUP: 636 – 6,990 ng/mg creatinine	328

*Buprenorphine (BUP), Norbuprenorphine (NBUP), Buprenorphine glucuronide (BUP-G), Norbuprenorphine glucuronide (NBUP-G).

When free buprenorphine was present at concentrations < 100 ng/mL (n=767) the mean ratio was 35.6 and the median 25.0. When free buprenorphine concentrations were ≥ 100 ng/mL and < 1000 ng/mL (n=19) the mean ratio was 0.30 and the median 0.15. In cases where free buprenorphine concentrations exceeded 1000 ng/mL, the mean ratio was 0.13 and the median 0.025 [352]. In pregnant patients, norbuprenorphine-glucuronide/buprenorphine-glucuronide ratios are significantly lower in the 2nd versus the 3rd trimester which is consistent with increased renal elimination, requiring higher daily doses during pregnancy [225].

After a single dose, buprenorphine has been detected in urine as quickly as 1 hour post-dose and norbuprenorphine in 2.5 hours [345]. The period of detection depends heavily on the method employed and testing thresholds. IA methods may not allow for periods of detection greater than 12 hours in many cases, whereas the period of detection for buprenorphine has been estimated to be up to four days based upon a single-dose study with LC/MS/MS analysis and a 0.5 ng/mL threshold for both buprenorphine and norbuprenorphine [334]. Buprenorphine use has been detected for up to 4-8 days with various methods [328, 334, 341].

Analysis of naloxone has been investigated for detection of buprenorphine/naloxone ingestion, though it is not usually performed in routine clinical testing. An estimated 24 – 37% of naloxone is excreted in urine within six hours, with very little excreted at 48 hours [388]. Following ingestion of buprenorphine/naloxone 16 mg/4 mg, 55% of the dose was excreted in the 24 hour urine as conjugated naloxone, unconjugated naloxone, and nornaloxone. The mean percentages of excreted daily dose were as follows: unconjugated naloxone 12.7%, conjugated naloxone 26.2%, unconjugated nornaloxone 6.4%, and conjugated nornaloxone 9.8% [56]. Sensitive testing techniques are required to detect naloxone in urine following sublingual buprenorphine administration, with reported limits of quantitation (LOQs) in the range of 0.1 – 10 ng/mL [56, 222].

Naloxone was undetectable in urine from patients maintained on sublingual buprenorphine/naloxone at a 100 ng/mL threshold [367]. However, this threshold lacked the sensitivity required to detect naloxone following ingestion of the buprenorphine combination product. Conversely, naloxone was detected in all samples of opioid dependence treatment patients at a LOQ of 1 ng/mL. The investigators suggest that if naloxone is not detected at this threshold it may suggest use of a buprenorphine-only product [222]. Free naloxone was not observed at LOQ 50 ng/mL in a subset of specimens with free buprenorphine < 20 ng/mL, free norbuprenorphine > 20 ng/mL, and glucuronides present, which is a typical pattern consistent with buprenorphine/naloxone ingestion. In a subset of specimens suspected for adulteration, free naloxone concentrations were relatively high [352]. These findings suggest adulteration attempts may be identified by assessing both buprenorphine and naloxone concentrations. Naloxone > 100 ng/mL may be indicative of buprenorphine administration through alternative routes such as intranasal or intravenous administration [329].

Naloxone concentrations (LOQ 1 ng/mL) and naloxone/buprenorphine ratios were assessed in patients undergoing maintenance treatment. Group 0 had not started maintenance treatment, Group 1 was in a stable treatment phase, and Group 2 was in an unstable phase of treatment. Overall, naloxone/buprenorphine ratios trended upward with increasing naloxone concentrations. The mean and median concentrations for each group (ng/mL), beginning with Group 0 were 57.1/0, 60.3/60, and 299.4/70. The concentration ranges (ng/mL) were 0 – 300, 5 – 200, and 10 – 1,700, respectively. The naloxone/buprenorphine ratio mean, median, and range were as follows (beginning with Group 0): 0.2/0 (0 – 1.0); 0.7/0.6 (0.05 – 2.6); 1.2/0.5 (0.06 – 8.9). Though the unstable Group 2 demonstrated the broadest range of concentrations, only 22% of the samples contained naloxone concentrations exceeding 200 ng/mL. Parenteral use of buprenorphine was associated with high naloxone/buprenorphine ratios. High ratios may also illustrate recent use as naloxone's half-life is shorter than buprenorphine [222].

Adulteration of urine specimens is common, due to attempts to cover illicit use or to falsify evidence of adherence to prescribed therapy. For this reason, it is advisable to conduct observed urine collections when policies and procedures allow [389]. Nearly 1 in 11 patients in addiction treatment were identified as having adulterated their urine specimens. Overall, 38% of patients submitted at least one suspicious sample (creatinine <20 mg/dL and/or norbuprenorphine/buprenorphine ratio < 0.02) [367]. SAMHSA guidelines classify specimens as dilute if creatinine is greater than 5 mg/dL but less than 20 mg/dL and specific gravity is equal to or greater than 1.002 but less than 1.003. Additionally, substitution is reported if creatinine is less than 2 mg/dL and specific gravity is less than or equal to 1.0010 or equal to or greater than 1.0200 [390]. Approximately 7% of specimens submitted to the Correctional Service of Canada over a period of two years were defined as dilute [391].

Patients engaging in diversion of their medications may attempt to appear compliant with prescribed medications by directly adding drug to urine post-collection. Such methods are difficult or impossible to detect by immunoassay, but parent and metabolite patterns discoverable following mass spectrometry testing may reveal anomalies suggestive of adulteration. Urine concentrations with high buprenorphine may be indicative of adulteration, particularly if metabolite is present at low concentrations or not detected [352, 367]. McMillin *et al.* concluded urine specimens containing > 100 ng/mL free buprenorphine in conjunction with low metabolite concentrations may be suggestive of adulteration; this impacted 4% of 1,946 urine specimens [352]. UDT results for patients indicate 1. 6 to 7.4% of specimens are positive for parent drug only in absence of metabolite [153, 370, 392]. In one study, 26.4% of parent-only results fell above the median concentration (73 ng/mL) of buprenorphine overall; the most common opioids found as parent-only were oxycodone, hydrocodone, buprenorphine, and fentanyl [392]. It should be noted that high concentrations alone do not necessarily support adulteration. Some patient specimens may contain greater amounts of buprenorphine than norbuprenorphine and lack characteristics indicative of adulteration [367]. Drug-drug interactions may influence excretion patterns. Even so, clinicians should consider metabolite patterns in the overall clinical context of the patient.

Very high concentrations of buprenorphine in absence of metabolites are concerning for adulteration and possible medication diversion. Interpretation may be complicated further when low concentrations of the metabolite norbuprenorphine are present. Buprenorphine concentrations between 1,000 – 100,000 ng/mL (abnormal for typical excretion) with low concentrations of metabolite are common and are strongly suggestive that norbuprenorphine may be present as a degradation product or impurity [392]. Other studies have demonstrated similar findings with minor concentrations of detectable norbuprenorphine in the presence of abnormally high concentrations of buprenorphine.

McMillin *et al.* found free norbuprenorphine to buprenorphine ratios between 0.00048 – 0.00397 and Hull *et al.* reported total norbuprenorphine/buprenorphine ratios < 0.02 (mean 0.009, SD=0.006) in samples for which adulteration was suspected [352, 367].

As discussed above, naloxone testing to pinpoint cases of adulteration has been suggested [352, 367]. Adulteration may be suggested by detection of free naloxone concentrations in urine; free naloxone concentrations were detected between 2,140 – 9,560 ng/mL, with corresponding buprenorphine/naloxone ratios of 3.5 to 4.5 [352].

Oral buprenorphine pharmaceutical preparations contain carbohydrates (e.g., disaccharides). These compounds break down in the small intestine to monosaccharides that are absorbed in the bloodstream when taken by intended route of ingestion. However, if buprenorphine products are ingested via alternatives routes such as injection, disaccharides may be detected in urine since they bypass breakdown in the gastrointestinal tract. In this way, the presence of disaccharides (e.g., lactose, sucrose) may be useful to detect adulteration or intravenous injection of buprenorphine. It is proposed these markers may be detectable for several hours. A significant number of specimens from intravenous abusers were found to be lactose positive (76.9%) and/or sucrose positive (73.1%). All patients in the control group were negative for disaccharides following ingestion of 20 grams each of sucrose and lactose.

Exceptions to this assessment may be prudent for patients with Crohn's disease or ulcerative colitis, as disaccharide absorption may occur through damaged small intestine [210]. Though urine testing for disaccharides is far from routine in clinical care, it does present an interesting opportunity worthy of further research.

ORAL FLUID

Oral fluid (primarily saliva) has been increasingly adopted as an alternative specimen for toxicology monitoring programs, and the ease of observed collection may be especially useful if urine adulteration or substitution is suspected [369, 393-396]. There are some important aspects to consider related to interpretation and testing methods. First, the oral fluid matrix necessitates higher technological requirements than urine analysis. Second, very high buprenorphine concentrations can lead to carryover problems affecting other oral fluid specimens during testing, particularly given low thresholds used. Laboratories should have steps in place to mitigate and assess for this occurrence. Third, proper collection is critical to decrease risk of contamination and assure adequate specimen volume collection. Prior to collection, it may be recommended that patients rinse their mouth with water, but 10 to 25 minutes should elapse prior to actual collection to allow drugs to re-equilibrate. This may not help reduce direct contamination in the cases of drug depot in the oral mucosa, as occurs with buprenorphine [381]. Fourth, the general period of detection for drugs in oral fluid is estimated to be 1 to 2 days for most analytes, which is shorter than urine [389].

The clinical buprenorphine threshold recommended by the United Kingdom National External Quality Assessment Service (UKNEQAS) is 5 ng/mL for oral fluid [397]. In a legal/treatment population, the thresholds for buprenorphine and norbuprenorphine were 1 ng/mL for IA and 0.5 ng/mL for GC/MS [398]. In pain management, buprenorphine ELISA thresholds of 2 ng/mL and 5 ng/mL have been used. LC/MS/MS thresholds have been reported as 0.5 – 2 ng/mL for buprenorphine and 1 – 2 ng/mL for norbuprenorphine [369, 395, 399].

A study by Cone *et al.* found 276 positives (3.4% positivity rate) for buprenorphine within a criminal justice intervention and/or rehabilitation population [398]. Similarly, a large study of more than 6,400 pain patients revealed a 2.6% positivity rate for buprenorphine [369]. Drug disposition differs from urine in that buprenorphine is generally the predominant analyte [369, 398-399]. In contrast to urine, buprenorphine-glucuronide and norbuprenorphine-glucuronide may be present in only 5% of oral fluid specimens at an LOQ of 0.6 ng/mL [380]. Norbuprenorphine can be very difficult to measure in oral fluid due to very low concentrations present, and published analytical methods vary in their inclusion of this metabolite [369, 381, 393, 395, 398]. In a criminal justice intervention and/or rehabilitation population, buprenorphine was detected in 95.3% and norbuprenorphine in

62.7% oral fluid specimens. Approximately 58% of specimens contained both analytes, whereas 37.3% and 4.7% contained buprenorphine-only and norbuprenorphine-only, respectively [398]. In pain management patients, buprenorphine was detected in 74% of specimens and norbuprenorphine in 48%. Buprenorphine-only was detected in 52% and norbuprenorphine-only in 26%; both analytes were detected in 22% of specimens submitted for analysis [369]. Acute dosing may result in buprenorphine concentrations exceeding norbuprenorphine, while buprenorphine may be less than or equal to norbuprenorphine in chronic use [400].

Oral fluid specimen concentrations in a criminal justice intervention and/or rehabilitation population ranged from 0.5 – 14,467 ng/mL (mean 433 ng/mL, median 24 ng/mL) for buprenorphine and 0.5 – 85 ng/mL (mean 5.0 ng/mL, median 2.0 ng/mL) for norbuprenorphine [398]. Buprenorphine concentrations ranging from 0.6 – 3,887 ng/mL (mean 140 – 240 ng/mL, median 16 – 32 ng/mL) have been reported in pain management patients with norbuprenorphine concentrations ranging from 2 – 196 ng/mL (mean 7 – 20 ng/mL, median 7 – 8 ng/mL). High buprenorphine concentrations are likely due to depot effect after sublingual administration [369, 394]. Chronic dosing of sublingual buprenorphine resulted in oral fluid concentrations ranging from 20 – 200 ng/mL 4 hours after administration [401]. Semi-quantitative buprenorphine concentrations in those undergoing sublingual substitution treatment (1 – 16 mg/day) were found to be 0.5 – 3.8 ng/mL [377].

Concentrations of buprenorphine and norbuprenorphine in oral fluid may be lower during pregnancy due to pharmacokinetic changes, though studies have revealed concentrations that should be readily detectable at conventional testing thresholds [380]. One patient receiving buprenorphine 16 mg SL daily had buprenorphine concentrations ranging from 0 – 7,400 ng/mL (median 170 ng/mL) and norbuprenorphine concentrations ranging from 0 – 71.3 ng/mL (median 4.1 ng/mL) [399]. In pregnant women receiving buprenorphine 14 – 20 mg SL, oral fluid concentrations ranges were as follows: buprenorphine 0.1 – 12,300 ng/mL and norbuprenorphine 0 – 55.6 ng/mL [380].

Comparisons of buprenorphine findings between oral fluid and urine, and oral fluid and blood have been published. Good overall agreement between oral fluid and urine was found through assessment of paired specimens in pain management patients. Buprenorphine was more likely to be detected in oral fluid and norbuprenorphine more likely to be detected in urine. Both analytes were detected simultaneously in some pairs [394]. Three paired specimens with low buprenorphine levels in urine <25 ng/mL were negative in oral fluid in another study, which may represent use several days prior to specimen collection [395]. Oral fluid concentrations are most closely related to plasma concentration, though correlations may be weak for some users [380, 389, 400]. Variability is observed depending on route of administration. Saliva/plasma (S:P) ratios < 1 may occur with intramuscular administration, likely due to high levels of plasma protein binding which can lead to low concentrations of buprenorphine in oral fluid [381, 400]. This is likely true for transdermal and subdermal administration as well; both formulations result in very low buprenorphine plasma concentrations in the subnanogram/mL range, resulting in unlikely detection of buprenorphine in oral fluid [8, 378, 395-396]. In contrast, the depot effect of sublingual buprenorphine can lead to very high drug concentrations [399-401]. S:P ratios may be > 1 following sublingual administration, with oral fluid concentrations more closely mirroring plasma levels by 24 to 48 hours post-dose [401]. At this time, oral fluid concentrations cannot be used to reliably estimate plasma concentrations, though positive findings may establish a closer relationship to impairment or clinical effect than urine concentrations.

Hair

Hair testing can provide historical information for up to 3 to 12 months of drug exposure depending on the segment analyzed, but is not utilized for assessment of recent use [389, 402]. Hair testing has been described in forensic cases but is not routinely used in clinical testing [309, 333]. It may take several weeks for buprenorphine and norbuprenorphine to be incorporated into hair for detection [328]. Hair is typically collected from the scalp, but other types of hair (e.g., axillary, pubic) have been used [389]. Hair pigment is an important factor affecting drug incorporation, with greater deposition of buprenorphine in pigmented hair than non-pigmented hair [328, 376, 403]. This effect can create a color bias during interpretation of results.

An additional confounding factor in hair testing interpretation is potential contamination resulting from environmental pollution. In postmortem cases, contamination due to sweat, putrefactive fluid, or blood may not be removed by washing, and may be suspected if concentrations are similar along the hair shaft regardless of segment location. The presence of metabolites does not rule out contamination, as they can also be present in contaminating materials [404]. Discrepancies between known period of drug use and predicted time frame of drug use in healthy subjects (based on hair analysis) have been observed, further supporting the theory that drug disposition in hair may be influenced by diffusion in sweat [376].

Hair testing methods do not universally include washing procedures. Predictably, higher drug concentrations have been detected in unwashed versus washed hair [405]. Washing/decontamination procedures have caused losses of buprenorphine and norbuprenorphine, with preferential losses of buprenorphine [406]. Interestingly, Goodwin *et al.* did not report significantly different norbuprenorphine/buprenorphine ratios between washed/unwashed specimens [405].

Degradation of buprenorphine/norbuprenorphine can take place rapidly and drug concentrations may be underestimated if acidic procedures are used to recover analytes [407]. Associations between dose and concentrations of buprenorphine/norbuprenorphine in washed and unwashed hair have been found [405]. Ratios of norbuprenorphine to buprenorphine have been shown to decrease distally along the hair shaft, indicating norbuprenorphine may be less tightly bound to hair than buprenorphine. Norbuprenorphine may be more susceptible to loss from hygienic care, greater adsorption from sweat, or weathering [405, 407].

The following methods have been described for hair analysis: CEDIA immunoassay, high performance liquid chromatography-electron detection (HPLC-ED), high performance liquid chromatography/mass spectrometry (HPLC/MS), HPLC/MS/MS, LC/MS/MS, and GC/MS. Reported thresholds and LOQs for buprenorphine and norbuprenorphine are several fold lower than LOQs used for urine, and have ranged from 3 – 50 pg/mg [328, 376, 385, 402, 405, 407-411].

Disposition of norbuprenorphine exceeds buprenorphine in hair of chronic users, with norbuprenorphine/buprenorphine ratios typically greater than one [328, 376, 406]. One study found ratios greater than three in all but one user of sublingual 8 mg in chronic treatment [376]. Variation exists and buprenorphine users will sometimes exhibit norbuprenorphine/buprenorphine ratios less than 1 [144, 309, 328, 406, 409]. High inter-subject variability also exists in terms of expected concentrations in hair [376]. In chronic treatment, buprenorphine concentrations have ranged from 0.8 – 2,360 pg/mg and norbuprenorphine concentrations from 4.8 – 2,018 pg/mg [328, 376, 405-407, 410, 412].

In overdoses, buprenorphine concentrations have ranged from 6 – 1,080 pg/mg and norbuprenorphine concentrations from 0 – 150 pg/mg [144, 298, 309, 377, 409].

SWEAT

Technologic requirements for sweat testing exceed those necessary for urine drug testing and sensitivity requirements are high [389]. Drugs enter sweat through two primary mechanisms: passive diffusion from blood to sweat glands (particularly for lipophilic drugs) and transdermal migration through the stratum corneum [413-414]. There is some concern regarding the potential for surface contamination as well and cleansing procedures should be implemented before patch application. Basic analytes may accumulate in sweat from blood due to pH differences between matrices [414]. SAMHSA has proposed sweat as a backup matrix for follow-up testing or treatment programs [415]. Periods of detection are generally expected to be similar to urine and limited to days in most cases [414]. LC/MS/MS (LOQ 1 ng/patch) and LC-ion spray MS (LOQ 0.2 ng/patch) methods have been described for testing of buprenorphine [415].

To collect sweat, a patch is typically worn for several days to a one-week period over which drugs accumulate, though two-week collections have been described [389, 414]. Patches resemble a large Band-Aid which is applied to the back, upper arm, or lower chest areas. They generally adhere well with little irritation [415]. However, in a study by Chawarski *et al.,* only 188 of 536 patches were properly worn and unadulterated. Many study subjects reported their patches had fallen off; these patches were not included in analysis given potential for environmental contamination or adulteration [413]. Improperly worn patches may impede effective monitoring in clinical settings.

High inter- and intra-subject variability is to be expected with sweat testing and no dose-concentration relationship has been established [389, 415-416]. This may be explained in part by differences in sweat excretion [416]. In general, parent drug concentrations exceed those of metabolites due to greater lipophilicity; this pattern has been observed for buprenorphine [415].

Buprenorphine detection in sweat has been reported for 16 – 75% of patients on maintenance therapy [380, 415]. In subjects receiving opioid-dependence treatment (0.4 – 6 mg SL/day) concentrations of buprenorphine were 1.3 – 153.2 ng/patch. Norbuprenorphine was only detected in one case at a concentration of 3.2 ng/patch, which coincided with the highest buprenorphine concentration [416]. In a study of pregnant women receiving buprenorphine 14 – 20 mg SL, buprenorphine was found from 1 – 2.3 ng/patch (median 1 ng/patch) and norbuprenorphine from 1 – 2.4 ng/patch [380, 415]. Many applications for sweat testing have focused on illicit drugs and methods for some of the more common drugs employed in pain management have not been described, including hydrocodone, oxycodone, alprazolam, clonazepam, and lorazepam [417]. This limitation, combined with the more limited detection rates in patients prescribed buprenorphine for maintenance treatment, may limit routine testing of sweat as part of compliance monitoring in clinical settings.

BREATH

Breath analysis for detection of drugs is a new technology under current development. Testing methodologies require ultra-sensitive procedures. Although its strengths and limitations have not been fully defined, its exploration seems worthwhile. Exhaled breath contains bioaerosol particles which are formed deep in lungs from non-volatile substances. Several exogenous substances, including drugs, have been identified in breath [418-419]. Understandably, breath analysis may identify drugs that have been smoked or inhaled, due to contamination of the airways (e.g., marijuana) [418]. The airway lining, consisting of proteins and lipids, may also act as its own distribution compartment for drugs that are not inhaled but rather distributed from blood. Breath specimens have demonstrated positive results for approximately 24 hours following drug ingestion, despite rapid turn-over rate [418-419]. Prior to breath specimen collection, the mouth should be rinsed [418]. Breath is exhaled through a mouthpiece which separates large particles from micro-particles, which are collected on polymer filter. Approximately 20 liters of exhaled breath can be collected in 2-3 minutes. One of the challenges faced in breath collection is standardization of collection procedures for quantitative applications [419]. In a study of eight patients presenting with acute intoxication, buprenorphine was detected in all patients with positive findings in urine or plasma, but three concentrations were below the 6 pg/filter LOQ. Breath concentrations ranged from 114 – 567 pg/filter and plasma concentrations from 162 – 333 ng/mL [419]. In a separate study of six patients presenting with acute intoxication with buprenorphine confirmed in plasma, buprenorphine was detected in breath in four cases at a LOQ of 0.08 pg/column, with concentrations ranging from 1.8 – 41 pg/min [418]. A breath/urine comparison study detected breath concentrations of 8 – 42 pg/filter (median 26 pg/filter), with breath selected as the preferred matrix of prison inmates and staff [420]. At this time, norbuprenorphine detection in breath has not been described and there is limited information regarding interpretive considerations, but breath analysis will almost certainly be an area of current and future study for various applications.

Other Specimens

Buprenorphine undergoes extensive distribution and other matrices such as bile, liver, brain, kidney, and myocardium have been used for drug detection in forensic applications. For example, high concentrations have been detected in bile, with buprenorphine concentrations ranging from 575 – 72,650 ng/mL and norbuprenorphine from 41 – 30,000 ng/mL [144]. Concentration data for buprenorphine and norbuprenorphine in various matrices more routinely used in clinical applications are summarized in Table 4.

Table 4. Buprenorphine concentrations in oral fluid, plasma, hair, sweat, and breath

Specimen Type	Concentrations*	References
Oral Fluid	BUP: 0.5-14,467 ng/mL NBUP: 0.5-196 ng/mL	369, 394, 398
Plasma	BUP: 0.7-56.0 ng/mL NBUP: 0.1-3.5 ng/mL	26, 34, 421-424
Hair	BUP: 0.8-2,360 pg/mg NBUP: 4.8-2,019 pg/mg	328, 376, 405-407, 410, 412, 425
Sweat	BUP: 1.3-153.2 ng/patch NBUP: 1-3.2 ng/patch	380, 415-416
Breath	BUP: 114 – 567 pg/filter	419

* Buprenorphine (BUP), norbuprenorphine (NBUP). Hydrolysis procedures were not necessarily applied in all cases of reported concentrations.

Neonatal Testing

Due to buprenorphine's increasing use in pregnant women for the treatment of opioid dependence, neonatal exposure has of course followed suit and testing of various biological matrices is of interest [218-219, 236-237, 239].

Drug exposure can affect fetal development and may have neurocognitive and physiological effects later in life, and detection of gestational exposure is a vital component of promoting child wellbeing [414, 426]. Identification of drug exposure is important for guiding neonatal treatment when NAS is present.

The average onset of withdrawal symptoms is similar to or exceeds the time to discharge of mother; for this reason, testing is a crucial component of identifying drug exposure when use is suspected, especially since maternal denial of drug use is common [427]. Various specimen types have been explored in neonatal testing aimed at identifying infant exposure to substances during the gestation period. There are unique characteristics and considerations for each matrix type.

Neonatal Testing: Blood

Buprenorphine and norbuprenorphine have described in neonatal serum, with higher buprenorphine concentrations found in the infant compared to the maternal trough prior to birth (1.9 vs 0.3 ng/mL) [31]. Ratios of buprenorphine/norbuprenorphine tend to be higher in neonates than in adults, which would be consistent with lower CYP3A4 metabolism of buprenorphine [428]. However, neonatal blood testing is not routinely performed.

Neonatal Testing: Urine

The highest infant urinary concentrations of norbuprenorphine have been demonstrated during the first three days after delivery, and were correlated with length of stay and duration of pharmacologic treatment for NAS. Despite this finding, a correlation for both factors could not be established on the basis of first day norbuprenorphine concentrations [429].

Urine concentrations may be 8 to 10-fold higher than blood concentrations, with norbuprenorphine expected as the predominant analyte [31, 118].

Urine buprenorphine neonatal concentrations have ranged from 1 to > 200 ng/mL and norbuprenorphine from 0 to > 200 ng/mL [31, 429]. Urine collection from neonates presents unique challenges not faced by the adult population, which has led to testing of alternative specimen matrices.

Neonatal Testing: Hair

Hair can serve as an option when urine and/or meconium are negative or not available. Neonatal hair testing reveals prenatal drug exposure in the last trimester due to maternal ingestion, as drugs are deposited from fetal blood or through contamination from amniotic fluid [427]. Hair testing of this type is qualitative and does not show degree of exposure [405]. In order for this specimen type to reveal exposure to maternal drug use during gestation, collection must occur during the first three months after delivery before infant hair replaces neonatal hair [427].

Washing procedures may not be used because the hair's fine texture may lead to excessive drug removal [405]. Testing of this matrix may be limited by insufficient hair quantity or the mother's objections for cosmetic or cultural reasons. An additional limitation relates to potential for pigmentation bias with basic drugs such as buprenorphine, which is a weak base with a pKa of 8.24 [30, 427].

Concentrations in neonatal hair tend to be present at concentrations 1 to 2 orders of magnitude higher than meconium. Typically, parent drugs are detected more readily in hair than metabolites [414]. Nonetheless, disposition of buprenorphine in neonatal hair appears to deviate from this pattern. Norbuprenorphine exceeds buprenorphine using a LOQ of 3 pg/mg for both analytes, with ratios of norbuprenorphine/buprenorphine ranging from 12.6 – 19.9.

Buprenorphine concentrations ranged from 37 – 82 pg/mg and norbuprenorphine ranged from 580 – 1,037 pg/mg. A statistically significant trend correlating buprenorphine concentrations in unwashed maternal and infant hair specimens has been observed; similar correlations could not be demonstrated for norbuprenorphine [405].

Neonatal Testing: Meconium

Meconium, a dark green/black odorless substance, is the first neonatal stool which is completely passed a few days following birth. It has been used to detect fetal exposure to illicit drugs [426]. Drugs and metabolites are incorporated into meconium by fetal biliary excretion or through swallowing drug-contaminated amniotic fluid. It starts forming at twelve weeks and consists of water, gastrointestinal and epithelial cells, lanugo, bile acids and salts, cholesterol and sterol precursors, blood group substances, enzymes, mucopolysaccharides, sugars, lipids, proteins, trace metals, pancreatic and intestinal secretions, and residue of swallowed amniotic fluid [426, 430]. Meconium has been increasingly used over last two decades. It has advantages over hair or urine due to an easier diaper collection process [426]. Urine collections are more difficult: the adhesive on the collection bag can irritate skin and it may come undone, leading to incomplete sample collection [431]. Meconium has consequently become the specimen of choice and is the most sensitive method for detecting drug exposure in neonates. Drug concentrations are also higher in meconium than urine due to accumulation [427]. Investigations into quantitation of drugs in meconium may help provide insight into correlations between fetal exposure and subsequent outcomes [430]. Concentrations of total buprenorphine in meconium and buprenorphine/norbuprenorphine ratios have been associated with diagnosable NAS, but not with requirement of pharmacotherapy [242]. Quantitation may not be useful in some cases because of contamination from urine [426].

Because meconium is a complex sample containing multiple compounds, it is difficult to isolate compounds, which can impede analysis [431]. Immunoassay, GC/MS, LC/MS/MS, and liquid chromatography/time-of-flight mass spectrometry (LC-TOFMS) methods have been described [426, 431]. Thresholds between 10 – 25 ng/g have been employed for detection of meconium buprenorphine and norbuprenorphine [426, 430-431]. A LC-TOFMS method with thresholds of 49 ng/g for norbuprenorphine and 18 ng/g for buprenorphine was compared to an LC/MS/MS method with lower thresholds of 5 ng/g for both buprenorphine and norbuprenorphine; the higher thresholds of the LC-TOFMS method resulted in detection of only 29% buprenorphine cases and 46% of norbuprenorphine cases [426]. Additionally, results observed with a 100 ng/g threshold with LC/MS/MS indicated greater sensitivity was necessary [431].

At least some analytical methods have difficulty incorporating buprenorphine with other analytes due to low concentrations present and the poor fragmentation profile of buprenorphine and norbuprenorphine, which lowers sensitivities and increases LOQs. Some investigators have used a second analytical run to quantify buprenorphine and norbuprenorphine separately, but sample volumes of meconium can be limited and this approach is not always practical [431]. Hydrolysis is not always used in meconium testing, and direct analysis of glucuronide conjugates has been described [430].

The period of detection for meconium testing is usually limited to the third trimester, but may potentially extend into the second trimester [426, 431].

Norbuprenorphine is the chief analyte in meconium. Fifteen percent of specimens in a study by Ristimaa *et al.* were positive for both buprenorphine and norbuprenorphine, 2% were positive for norbuprenorphine only, and none were positive for buprenorphine only [426]. Buprenorphine concentrations of 1.3 – 107 ng/g and norbuprenorphine up to 295 ng/g have been reported. Concentrations in meconium can increase with subsequent bowel movements. In one example, the first and third meconium sample concentrations of buprenorphine were 1.3 and 35.4 ng/g buprenorphine, respectively [31].

Neonatal Testing: Placenta

The placental membrane is thin and allows easy transfer of small lipophilic molecules, whereas transfer of hydrophilic molecules occurs at a slower rate [223]. Buprenorphine is rapidly perfused from maternal blood to the placenta within 1 hour. Although placental buprenorphine concentrations may be 20-fold higher than maternal blood concentrations, most buprenorphine is sequestered in the placenta and less than 10% is delivered to fetal circulation.

It is estimated that less than 5% of perfused buprenorphine is metabolized to norbuprenorphine [228]. LC/MS methods have been described in testing placenta [432]. Aromatase/CYP19 has been identified as the major enzyme responsible for conversion of buprenorphine to norbuprenorphine in placental tissue, beginning at 17 weeks gestation and increasing with gestational age [433-434]. UGTs exist in placenta but no data specific to buprenorphine metabolism are available [432]. Buprenorphine is not a substrate of the placental P-glycoprotein efflux transporter [435].

The period of detection for buprenorphine in placenta has been estimated to be at least one week. Norbuprenorphine and norbuprenorphine-glucuronide are the predominant analytes and placental concentrations are 15 to 70-fold lower than those in meconium. Buprenorphine, norbuprenorphine, buprenorphine-glucuronide, and norbuprenorphine-glucuronide concentrations have been published in the following ranges: 0 – 3.2 ng/g, 6.2 – 24.2 ng/g, 1.3 – 5.0 ng/g, and 11.4 – 46.6 ng/g [432, 436]. Numerous correlations for quantitative results have been observed including mean maternal daily dose and buprenorphine-glucuronide concentrations in placenta; norbuprenorphine-glucuronide concentrations and time to NAS onset and duration; and norbuprenorphine/norbuprenorphine-glucuronide ratios and maximum NAS score and newborn length [432].

Neonatal Testing: Umbilical Cord or Umbilical Cord Blood

Collection of umbilical cord or cord blood may be more easily accomplished than collection for other specimen types, thus increasing interest in clinical settings. Umbilical cord or cord blood testing reveals *in utero* drug exposure, with a longer window of detection for cord than for cord blood [427]. Generally there is low transfer to cord blood from the maternal compartment, with buprenorphine and norbuprenorphine cord blood to maternal ratios < 1, and mostly 0.5 or lower [379, 437]. Norbuprenorphine glucuronide has been shown to be the predominant metabolite. Gordon *et al.* reports buprenorphine was frequently undetected at a LOQ of 0.125 ng/mL [437]. Other studies have reported buprenorphine concentrations ranging from 0.1 – 0.5 ng/mL in cord blood [118, 379, 438]. Norbuprenorphine, buprenorphine glucuronide, and norbuprenorphine glucuronide concentrations have been reported as follows: 0.9 – 1.5 ng/mL, 4.6 ng/mL, and 29.8 ng/mL [379, 438].

Cord concentrations are similar to cord plasma concentrations, and it is likely that buprenorphine analytes passively diffuse into cord from plasma. Concentrations are lower in cord (16 to 210-fold) than meconium. Parent buprenorphine is often not detected and the following concentrations have been found for buprenorphine metabolites: norbuprenorphine 1.2 – 5.1 ng/g (mean 3.1, median 2.5 ng/g); buprenorphine glucuronide 1.7 – 4.2 ng/g (mean 3.0, median 3.0 ng/g); and norbuprenorphine glucuronide 8.3 – 23 ng/g (mean 17.3, median 18 ng/g). Correlations have not been established between umbilical cord concentrations and neonatal outcomes [439].

Conclusion

Buprenorphine has been used for many years internationally. Its use has been applied and investigated in various clinical scenarios, including opioid dependence treatment, detoxification, and pain management. While it may be viewed as a safer alternative to other opioids (including methadone) given its ceiling effect and decreased risk for respiratory depression, drug-drug interactions including concomitant use of CNS depressants may diminish safety advantages. Availability of abuse-deterrent formulations may make buprenorphine an appealing option for some patients, but abuse still occurs. Increasing rates of buprenorphine abuse and misuse have contributed to rises in drug overdoses and fatalities involving buprenorphine, particularly in conjunction with poly-substance use. When considering buprenorphine versus methadone in opioid dependence treatment, it is important to note neither is considered the gold standard in all patients and providers may have preferences for one over the other. The choice between buprenorphine and methadone should be tailored to the unique needs and medical/social history of each individual patient. Logistics regarding patient access to each therapy also may influence prescribing choice. In pregnant patients, buprenorphine has been explored as an alternative therapy to methadone and information in the literature describes buprenorphine as having a similar safety profile. Neonatal abstinence is less severe for buprenorphine-exposed infants than methadone, and further research is warranted to more clearly define its role in obstetric patients. Though there is a plethora of published information detailing buprenorphine properties and its clinical utility, there is a multitude of ongoing studies involving buprenorphine (registered in clinicaltrials.gov) investigating drug pharmacokinetics, drug-drug interactions, use in HIV populations, use in pregnancy and neonatal outcomes, buprenorphine-based treatment of NAS, strategies for the treatment of opioid dependence and pain management, and detoxification. Research discoveries will continue to shape buprenorphine's place in therapy in various populations.

While use of buprenorphine may lower mortality or morbidity relative to abuse of other drugs, unmonitored use/abuse can pose a danger to the patient. The high prevalence of benzodiazepine use (whether prescribed or non-prescribed) by patients ingesting buprenorphine is cause for concern. Inclusion of buprenorphine in toxicology testing should therefore be considered by providers in clinical settings. In pain management and opioid treatment populations, buprenorphine is often prescribed and patient compliance is important to assess given the propensity for misuse and abuse. Additionally, it may be considered an important component of toxicology testing profiles for patients not prescribed buprenorphine as well, given the increases in illicit use and NFLIS seizures of this drug over the past decade. Toxicology testing provides objective information that is a crucial component of overall patient assessment and has been described in many different matrices, including urine, oral fluid, blood, hair, and sweat. Urine and oral fluid testing are most commonly employed in clinical practice for buprenorphine; plasma concentrations may be low, and transdermal buprenorphine is unlikely to be detected in either blood or oral fluid at typical thresholds (>1 ng/mL). In neonatal populations, testing is usually performed with hair, urine, meconium, and umbilical cord or cord blood. Monitoring for buprenorphine presence in biological specimens can present analytical and interpretive challenges which may vary between matrices, and a basic knowledge of these differences is clearly useful in clinical practice.

ACKNOWLEDGMENT

The authors wish to thank Elizabeth Baker and Aegis Sciences Corporation for library services.

REFERENCES

[1] Baselt, R. C. Disposition of Toxic Drugs and Chemicals in Man. 9th Ed. Seal Beach, CA: Biomedical Publications; 2011.

[2] Johnson, R. E.; Fudala, P. J.; Payne, R. Buprenorphine: considerations for pain management. *J. Pain Symptom Manage*, 2005, 29(3), 297-326.

[3] Yokell, M. A.; Zaller, N. D.; Green, T. C.; et al. Buprenorphine and buprenorphine/naloxone diversion, misuse, and illicit use: an international review. *Curr. Drug Abuse Rev.*, 2011, 4, 28–41.

[4] Chen, K. Y.; Chen, L.; Mao, J. Buprenorphine-naloxone therapy in pain management. Anesthesiology, 2014, 120, epub ahead of print.

[5] Drug Enforcement Administration, Office of Diversion Control, Drug and Chemical Evaluation Section. Buprenorphine [online]. July 2013 [2014 February 16]. Available from: http:// www.deadiversion.usdoj.gov/drug_chem_info/buprenorphine.pdf

[6] Reckitt Benckiser Pharmaceuticals, Inc. Suboxone prescribing information. Richmond, VA. August 2012.

[7] Comer, S. D.; Sullivan, M. A.; Vosburg, S. K.; et al. Abuse liability of intravenous buprenorphine/naloxone and buprenorphine alone in buprenorphine maintained intravenous heroin abusers. *Addiction*, 2010, 105, 709-18.

[8] Purdue Pharma L. P. Butrans prescribing information. Stamford, C. T., July 2012.

[9] Belcheva, M. M.; Barg, J.; McHale, R. J.; et al. Differential down- and up-regulation of rat brain opioid receptor types and subtypes by buprenorphine. *Mol. Pharmacol.*, 1993, 44, 173–9.

[10] Negus, S. S.; Bidlack, J. M.; Mello, N. K.; et al. Delta opioid antagonist effects of buprenorphine in rhesus monkeys. *Behav. Pharmacol.*, 2002, 13, 557–70.

[11] Bloms-Funke, P.; Gillen, C.; Schuettler, A. J.; et al. Agonistic effects of the opioid buprenorphine on the nociceptin/OFQ receptor. *Peptides*, 2000, 21, 1141–6.

[12] Herz, A. Opioid reward mechanisms: a key role in drug abuse? *Can. J. Physiol. Pharmacol.*, 1998, 76, 252-8.

[13] Cowan, A.; Lewis, J. W.; MacFarlane, I. R. Agonist and antagonist properties of buprenorphine, a new antinociceptive agent. *Br. J. Pharmacol.,* 1977, 60, 537–45.

[14] Tyers, M. B. A classification of opiate receptors that mediate antinociception in animals. *Br. J. Pharmacol.*, 1980, 69, 503-12.

[15] Dum, J. E.; Herz, A. In vivo receptor binding of the opiate partial agonist, buprenorphine, correlated with its agonistic and antagonistic actions. *Br. J. Pharmacol.*, 1981, 74, 627–33.

[16] Sadée, W.; Rosenbaum, J.; Herz, A. Buprenorphine: differential interaction with opiate receptor subtypes in vivo. *J. Pharmacol. Exp. Ther.*, 1982, 223, 157–62.

[17] Pick, C. G.; Peter, Y.; Schreiber, S.; et al. Pharmacological characterization of buprenorphine, a mixed agonist-antagonist with k3 analgesia. *Brain Res.,* 1997, 744, 41– 6.

[18] Lutfy, K.; Eitan, S.; Bryant, C. D.; et al. Buprenorphine-induced antinociception is mediated by μ-opioid receptors and compromised by concomitant activation of opioid receptor-like receptors. *J. Neurosci.,* 2003, 23, 10331–7.

[19] Hayes, A. G.; Sheehan, M. J.; Tyers, M. B. Differential sensitivity of models of antinociception in the rat, mouse and guinea-pig to μ- and κ-opioid receptor agonists. *Br. J. Pharmacol.*, 1987, 91, 823–32.

[20] Greenwald, M. K.; Johanson, C. E.; Moody, D. E.; et al. Effects of buprenorphine maintenance dose on μ-opioid receptor availability, plasma concentrations, and antagonist blockade in heroin-dependent volunteers. *Neuropsychopharmacology*, 2003, 28, 2000–9.

[21] Fudala, P. J.; Jaffe, J. H.; Dax, E. M.; et al. Use of buprenorphine in the treatment of opioid addiction. II. Physiologic and behavioral effects of daily and alternate-day administration and abrupt withdrawal. *Clin. Pharmacol. Ther.*, 1990, 47, 525–34.

[22] Eissenberg, T.; Greenwald, M. K.; Johnson, R. E.; et al. Buprenorphine's physical dependence potential: antagonist-precipitated withdrawal in humans. *J. Pharmacol. Exp. Ther.*, 1996, 276, 449–59.

[23] Boas, R. A.; Villiger, J. W. Clinical actions of fentanyl and buprenorphine. The significance of receptor binding. *Br. J. Anaesth.*, 1985, 57, 192–6.

[24] Walsh, S. L.; Stoller, K. L.; Bigelow, G. E.; et al. Acute administration of buprenorphine in humans: partial agonist and blockade effects. *Journal of Pharmacology and Experimental Therapeutics*, 1995, 274, 361–72.

[25] Bullingham, R. E. S.; McQuay, H. J.; Porter, E. J. B.; et al. Sublingual buprenorphine used postoperatively: ten hour plasma drug concentration analysis. *Br. J. Clin. Pharmacol.*, 1982, 13, 665–73.

[26] Kuhlman, J. J.; Lalani, S., Magluilo, J.; et al. Human pharmacokinetics of intravenous, sublingual, and buccal buprenorphine. *J. Anal. Toxicol.,* 1996, 20(6), 369–78.

[27] Iribarne, C.; Picart, D.; Dréano, Y.; et al. Involvement of cytochrome P450 3A4 in N-dealkylation of buprenorphine in human liver microsomes. *Life Sci.,* 1997, 60, 1953-64.

[28] Helm, S.; Trescot, A. M.; Colson, J.; et al. Opioid antagonists, partial agonists, and agonists/antagonists: the role of office-based detoxification. *Pain Physician*, 2008, 11(2), 225-35.

[29] Compton, P.; Ling, W.; Chiang, N.; et al. Pharmacokinetics of buprenorphine: a comparison of sublingual tablet versus liquid after chronic dosing. *J. Addict Med.,* 2007, 1(2), 88-95.

[30] Mendelson, J.; Upton, R. A.; Everhart, E. T.; et al. Bioavailability of sublingual buprenorphine. *J. Clin. Pharmacol.*, 1997, 37, 31–7.

[31] Elkader, A.; Sproule, B. Buprenorphine: clinical pharmacokinetics in the treatment of opioid dependence. *Clin. Pharmacokinet.*, 2005, 44 (7), 661–80.

[32] Walsh, S. L.; Preston, K. L.; Stitzer, M. L.; et al. Clinical pharmacology of buprenorphine: ceiling effects at high doses. *Clin. Pharmacol. Ther.*, 1994, 55, 569–80.

[33] Schuh, K. J.; Johanson, C. E. Pharmacokinetic comparison of the buprenorphine sublingual liquid and tablet. *Drug Alcohol Depend.*, 1999, 56(1), 55-60.

[34] Harris, D. S.; Mendelson, J.E.; Lin, E. T.; et al. Pharmacokinetics and subjective effects of sublingual buprenorphine, alone or in combination with naloxone. *Clin. Pharmacokinet.*, 2004, 43(5), 329-40.

[35] Chiang, C. N.; Hawks, R. L. Pharmacokinetics of the combination tablet of buprenorphine and naloxone. *Drug Alcohol Depend.*, 2003, S39-47.

[36] Umbricht, A.; Huestis, M. A.; Cone, E. J.; et al. Effects of high-dose intravenous buprenorphine in experienced opioid abusers. *J. Clin. Psychopharmacol.*, 2004, 24(5), 479–87.

[37] Kapil, R. P.; Cipriano, A.; Friedman, K.; et al. Once-weekly transdermal buprenorphine application results in sustained and consistent steady-state plasma levels. *J. Pain Symptom Manage,* 2013, 46(1), 65-75.

[38] Eriksen, J.; Jensen, N. H.; Kamp-Jensen, M.; et al. The systemic availability of buprenorphine administered by nasal spray. *J. Pharm. Pharmacol.,* 1989, 41, 803–5.

[39] Middleton, L. S.; Nuzzo, P. A.; Lofwall, M. R.; et al. The pharmacodynamic and pharmacokinetic profile of intranasal crushed buprenorphine and buprenorphine/naloxone tablets in opioid abusers. *Addiction*, 2011, 106, 1460–73.

[40] Hussain, A. A. Nasal absorption of naloxone and buprenorphine in rats. *Int. J. Pharm.*, 1984, 21, 233-7.

[41] Orman, J. S., Keating, G. M. Buprenorphine/naloxone: a review of its use in the treatment of opioid dependence. *Drugs,* 2009, 69(5), 577–607.

[42] Merlin, M. A.; Saybolt, M.; Kapitanyan, R.; et al. Intranasal naloxone delivery is an alternative to intravenous naloxone for opioid overdoses. *Am. J. Emerg. Med.*, 2010, 28, 296-303.

[43] Pontani, R. B.; Vadlamani, N. L.; Misra, A. L. Disposition in the rat of buprenorphine administered parenterally and as a subcutaneous implant. *Xenobiotica*, 1985, 15, 287–97.

[44] Ohtani, M.; Kotaki, H.; Sawada, Y.; et al. Comparative analysis of buprenorphine- and norbuprenorphine-induced analgesic effects based on pharmacokinetic-pharmacodynamic modeling. *J. Pharmacol. Exp. Ther.*, 1995, 272, 505-10.

[45] Ohtani, M. Basic pharmacology of buprenorphine. *Eur. J. Pain Suppl.,* 2007, 1, 69–73.

[46] Harris, D. S.; Jones, R. T.; Welm, S.; et al. Buprenorphine and naloxone co-administration in opiate-dependent patients stabilized on sublingual buprenorphine. *Drug Alcohol Depend.*, 2000, 61, 85–94.

[47] Cone, E. J.; Gorodetzky, C. W.; Yousefnejad, D.; et al. The metabolism and excretion of buprenorphine in humans. *Drug Metab. Dispos.*, 1984, 12, 577-81.

[48] Moody, D. E.; Slawson, M. H.; Strain, E. C.; et al. A liquid chromatographic-electrospray ionization-tandem mass spectrometric method for determination of buprenorphine, its metabolite, norbuprenorphine, and a co-formulant, naloxone, that is suitable for in vivo and in vitro metabolism studies. *Anal. Biochem.*, 2002, 306, 31-9.

[49] Moody, D. E.; Chang, Y.; Huang, W.; et al. The in vivo response of novel buprenorphine metabolites, M1 and M3, to antiretroviral inducers and inhibitors of buprenorphine metabolism. *Basic Clin. Pharmacol. Toxicol.*, 2009, 105(3), 211-5.

[50] Picard, N.; Cresteil, T.; Djebli, N.; et al. In vitro metabolism study of buprenorphine: evidence for new metabolic pathways. *Drug Metab. Dispos.*, 2005, 33(5), 689-95.

[51] Chang, Y.; Moody, D. E.; McCance-Katz, E. F. Novel metabolites of buprenorphine detected in human liver microsomes and human urine. *Drug Metab. Dispos.*, 2006, 34(3), 440-8.

[52] Rouguieg, K.; Picard, N.; Sauvage, F. L.; et al. Contribution of the different UDP-glucuronosyltransferase (UGT) isoforms to buprenorphine and norbuprenorphine metabolism and relationship with the main UGT polymorphisms in a bank of human liver microsomes. *Drug Metab. Dispos.*, 2010, 38, 40-5.

[53] Brown, S. M.; Holtzman, M.; Kim, T.; et al. Buprenorphine metabolites, buprenorphine-3-glucuronide and norbuprenorphine-3-glucuronide, are biologically active. *Anesthesiology*, 2011, 115, 1251–60.

[54] Moody, D. E.; Fang, W. B.; Morrison, J.; et al. Gender differences in pharmacokinetics of maintenance dosed buprenorphine. *Drug Alcohol Depend.*, 2011, 118(2-3), 479-83.

[55] Lalovic, B.; Phillips, B.; Risler, L. L.; et al. Quantitative contribution of CYP2D6 and CYP3A to oxycodone metabolism in human liver and intestinal microsomes. *Drug Metab. Dispos.*, 2004, 32, 447-54.

[56] Fang, W. B.; Chang, Y.; McCance-Katz, E. F.; et al. Determination of naloxone and nornaloxone (noroxymorphone) by high-performance liquid-chromatography-electrospray ionization-tandem mass spectrometry. *J. Anal. Toxicol.*, 2009, 33(8), 409-17.

[57] Weinstein, S. H.; Pfeffer, M.; Schor, J. M. Metabolism and pharmacokinetics of naloxone. *Adv. Biochem. Psychopharmacol.*, 1974, 8, 525–35.

[58] Ohtani, M.; Kotaki, H.; Uchino, K.; et al. Pharmacokinetic analysis of enterohepatic circulation of buprenorphine and its active metabolite, norbuprenorphine, in rats. *Drug Metab. Dispos.*, 1994, 22(1), 2-7.

[59] Seldén, T.; Ahlner, J.; Druid, H.; et al. Toxicological and pathological findings in a series of buprenorphine related deaths. Possible risk factors for fatal outcome. *Forensic Sci. Int.*, 2012, 220, 284-90.

[60] Wolters Kluwer Health. Facts and Comparisons® eAnswers [online]. 2013 [2013 December 12]. Available from: http://online.factsandcomparisons.com/index.aspx

[61] Reckitt Benckiser Pharmaceuticals, Inc. Discontinuation of sale and distribution of Subutex® tablets CIII. Press release [online]. September 16, 2011 [2014 February 14]. Available from: http://buprenorphine.samhsa.gov/SubutexDiscontinuation9-16-11.pdf

[62] Reckitt Benckiser Pharmaceuticals, Inc. Questions and answers about the discontinuation of Suboxone® (buprenorphine and naloxone) sublingual tablet (CIII) [online]. January 10, 2013 [2014 February 27]. Available from: http://www.suboxone.com

[63] JBS International, Inc. Diversion and abuse of buprenorphine: a brief assessment of emerging indicators: final report. Substance Abuse and Mental Health Services Administration Center for Substance Abuse Treatment, Silver Spring, MD, 2006.

[64] Orexo U. S., Inc. Zubsolv prescribing information. New York, NY, 2013.

[65] Reckitt Benckiser Pharmaceuticals, Inc. Reckitt Benckiser Pharmaceuticals Inc. receives FDA approval for Suboxone® (buprenorphine and naloxone) sublingual film C-III. Press release [online]. August 31, 2010 [2014 February 26]. Available at: http://www.rb.com/fda-approval-for-suboxone-sublingual-filmc-iii

[66] Lintzeris, N.; Leung, S. Y.; Dunlop, A. J.; et al. A randomised controlled trial of sublingual buprenorphine-naloxone film versus tablets in the management of opioid dependence. *Drug Alcohol Depend.*, 2013, 131(1-2), 119-26.

[67] Pontani, R. B.; Misra, A. L. A long-acting buprenorphine delivery system. *Pharmacol. Biochem. Behav.*, 1983, 18(3), 471-4.

[68] Titan Pharmaceuticals, Inc. Products and technologies: Probuphine® [online]. 2014 [2014, February 13]. Available from: http://www.titanpharm.com/products.htm

[69] Ling, W.; Casadonte, P.; Bigelow, G.; et al. Buprenorphine implants for treatment of opioid dependence: a randomized controlled trial. *JAMA,* 2010, 304(14), 1576-83.

[70] Titan Pharmaceuticals, Inc. Titan Pharmaceuticals receives complete response letter from the FDA for Probuphine new drug application. Press Release [online]. April 30, 2013 [2013 December 12]. Available from: http://www.titanpharm.com/press/2013/13-04-30-Titan-CRL.htm

[71] Mendelson, J.; Jones, R. T.; Welm, S.; et al. Buprenorphine and naloxone combinations: the effects of three dose ratios in morphine-stabilized, opiate-dependent volunteers. *Psychopharmacology,* 1999, 141, 37–46.

[72] Comer, S. D.; Collins, E. D. Self-administration of intravenous buprenorphine and the buprenorphine/naloxone combination by recently detoxified heroin abusers. *J. Pharmacol. Exp. Ther.,* 2002, 303(2), 695–703.

[73] Preston, K. L.; Bigelow, G. E.; Liebson, I. A. Buprenorphine and naloxone alone and in combination in opioid dependent humans. *Psychopharmacology*, 1988, 94, 484–90.

[74] Mendelson, J.; Jones, R. T.; Fernandez, I.; et al. Buprenorphine and naloxone interactions in opiate-dependent volunteers. *Clin. Pharmacol. Ther.*, 1996, 60, 105–14.

[75] Fudala, P. J.; Yu, E.; Macfadden, W.; et al. Effects of buprenorphine and naloxone in morphine-stabilized opioid addicts. *Drug Alcohol Depend.,* 1998, 50, 1–8.

[76] Stoller, K. B.; Bigelow, G. E.; Walsh, S. L.; et al. Effects of buprenorphine/naloxone in opioid-dependent humans. *Psychopharmacology,* 2001, 154, 230–42.

[77] Simojoki, K.; Vorma, H.; Alho, H. A retrospective evaluation of patients switched from buprenorphine (Subutex) to the buprenorphine/naloxone combination (Suboxone). *Subst. Abuse Treat. Prev. Policy*, 2008, 3(16), 1-6.

[78] Fudala, P. J.; Bridge, T. P.; Herbert, S.; et al. Office-based treatment of opiate addiction with a sublingual-tablet formulation of buprenorphine and naloxone. *N. Engl. J. Med.*, 2003, 349(10), 949-58.

[79] Daulouède, J. P.; Caer, Y.; Galland, P.; et al. Preference for buprenorphine/naloxone and buprenorphine among patients receiving buprenorphine maintenance therapy in France: a prospective, multicenter study. *J. Subst. Abuse Treat.*, 2010, 38(1), 83-9.

[80] Lange, W. R.; Fudala, P. J.; Dax, E. M.; et al. Safety and side-effects of buprenorphine in the clinical management of heroin addiction. *Drug Alcohol Depend.*, 1990, 26, 19–28.

[81] Dahan, A.; Yassen, A.; Bijl, H.; et al. Comparison of the respiratory effects of intravenous buprenorphine and fentanyl in humans and rats. *Br. J. Anaesth.*, 2005, 94, 825–34.

[82] Dahan, A.; Yassen, A.; Romberg, R.; et al. Buprenorphine induces ceiling in respiratory depression but not in analgesia. *Br. J. Anaesth.*, 2006, 96, 627–32.

[83] Dahan, A. Opioid-induced respiratory effects: new data on buprenorphine. *Palliat. Med.*, 2006, 20, s3-8.

[84] Huestis, M. A.; Cone, E. J.; Pirnay, S. O.; et al. Intravenous buprenorphine and norbuprenorphine pharmacokinetics in humans. *Drug Alcohol Depend.*, 2013, 131(3), 258-62.

[85] Huestis, M. A.; Umbitch, A.; Preston, K. L.; et al. Safety of buprenorphine: no clinically relevant cardio-respiratory depression at high IV doses. *NIDA Res. Monogr.*, 1999, 179, 62.

[86] Mégarbane, B.; Marie, N.; Pirnay, S.; et al. Buprenorphine is protective against the depressive effects of norbuprenorphine on ventilation. *Toxicol. Appl. Pharmacol.*, 2006, 212, 256–67.

[87] Heel, R. C.; Brogden, R. N.; Speight, T. M.; et al. Buprenorphine: a review of its pharmacological properties and therapeutic efficacy. *Drugs,* 1979, 17(2), 81-110.

[88] Downing, J. W.; Goodwin, N. M.; Hicks, J. The respiratory depressive effects of intravenous buprenorphine in patients in an intensive care unit. *S. Afr. Med. J.*, 1979, 55, 1023–7.

[89] Ohtani, M.; Kotaki, H.; Nishitateno, K.; et al. Kinetics of respiratory depression in rats induced by buprenorphine and its metabolite norbuprenorphine. *J. Pharmacol. Exp. Ther.*, 1997, 281, 428–33.

[90] Gueye, P. N.; Borron, S. W.; Risède, P.; et al. Lack of effect of single high doses of buprenorphine on arterial blood gases in the rat. *Toxicol. Sci.*, 2001, 62, 148–54.

[91] Knape, J. T. Early respiratory depression resistant to naloxone following epidural buprenorphine. *Anesthesiology,* 1986, 64, 382–4.

[92] Pedapati, E. V.; Bateman, S. T. Toddlers requiring pediatric intensive care unit admission following at-home exposure to buprenorphine/naloxone. *Pediatr. Crit. Care Med.*, 2011, 12(2), e102–7.

[93] Bickel, W. K.; Stitzer, M. L.; Bigelow, G. E.; et al. Buprenorphine: dose related blockade of opioid challenge effects in opioid dependent humans *J. Pharmacol. Exp. Ther.,* 1988, 247, 47–53.

[94] Center for Substance Abuse Treatment. Clinical Guidelines for the Use of Buprenorphine in the Treatment of Opioid Addiction. Treatment Improvement Protocol (TIP) Series 40. DHHS Publication No. (SMA) 04-3939. Rockville, MD: Substance Abuse and Mental Health Services Administration, 2004.

[95] Gruber, V. A.; McCance-Katz, E. F. Methadone, buprenorphine, and street drug interactions with antiretroviral medications. *Curr. HIV/AIDS Rep.,* 2010, 7(3), 152-60.

[96] Jasinski, D. R.; Pevnick, J. S.; Griffith, J. D. Human pharmacology and abuse potential of the analgesic buprenorphine. *Arch. Gen. Psychiatry,* 1978, 35, 501-16.

[97] Strain, E. C.; Preston, K. L.; Liebson, I. A.; et al. Buprenorphine effects in methadone-maintained volunteers: effects at two hours after methadone. *J. Pharmacol. Exp. Ther*., 1995, 272, 628–38.

[98] Walsh, S. L.; June, H. L.; Schuh, K. J.; et al. Effects of buprenorphine and methadone in methadone-maintained subjects. *Psychopharmacology,* 1995, 119, 268-76.

[99] Kögel, B.; Christoph, T.; Straßburger, W.; et al. Interaction of μ-opioid receptor agonists and antagonists with the analgesic effect of buprenorphine in mice. *Eur. J. Pain*, 2005, 9, 599-611.

[100] Heit H. A.; Gourlay D. L. Buprenorphine – new tricks with an old molecule for pain management. *Clin. J. Pain*, 2008, 24, 93-7.

[101] Johnson, R. E.; Strain, E. C.; Amass, L. Buprenorphine: how to use it right. *Drug Alcohol Depend.*, 2003, 70, S59–77.

[102] Wala, E. P.; Holtman Jr., J. R. Buprenorphine-induced hyperalgesia in the rat. *Eur. J. Pharmacol.*, 2011, 651(1-3), 89-95.

[103] Daitch, J.; Frey, M.; Silver, D.; et al. Conversion of chronic pain patients from full-opioid agonists to sublingual buprenorphine. *Pain Physician,* 2012, 15(3 Suppl.), ES59-66.

[104] Takahashi, T.; Okubo, K.; Kojima, S.; et al. Antihyperalgesic effect of buprenorphine involves nociception/orphanin FQ peptide-receptor activation in rats with spinal nerve injury-induced neuropathy. *J. Pharmacol. Sci.*, 2013, 122(1), 51-4.

[105] Compton, P.; Canamar, C. P.; Hillhouse, M.; et al. Hyperalgesia in heroin dependent patients and the effects of opioid substitution therapy. *J. Pain*, 2012, 13(4), 401-9.

[106] Masson, C. L.; Rainey, P. M.; Moody, D. E.; et al. Effects of HCV seropositive status on buprenorphine pharmacokinetics in opioid-dependent individuals. *Am. J. Addict*, 2014, 23(1), 34-40.

[107] Yee, A.; Loh, H. S.; Hisham Hashim, H. M.; et al. The prevalence of sexual dysfunction among male patients on methadone and buprenorphine treatments: a meta-analysis study. *J. Sex. Med.*, 2014, 11(1), 22-32.

[108] Smith, H. S.; Elliott, J. A. Opioid-induced androgen deficiency. *Pain Physician,* 2012, 15, ES145-56.

[109] Delgado-Charro, M. B.; Guy, R. H. Effective use of transdermal drug delivery in children. *Adv. Drug Deliv. Rev.,* 2013, Dec 11. pii: S0169-409X(13)00286-X. doi: 10.1016/j.addr.2013.11.014. [Epub ahead of print]

[110] Mundipharma Pharmaceuticals Limited. Transtec transdermal patch prescribing information. Dublin, Ireland, July 2012.

[111] Al-Tawil, N.; Odar-Cederlöf, I.; Berggren, A. C.; et al. Pharmacokinetics of transdermal buprenorphine patch in the elderly. *Eur. J. Clin. Pharmacol.*, 2013, 69(2), 143-9.

[112] Srinivas, N. R. Transdermal buprenorphine – interesting observations on the metabolite norbuprenorphine levels in elderly subjects. *Eur. J. Clin. Pharmacol.*, 2013, 69(8), 1607-8.

[113] Karlsson, J.; Söderström, A.; Augustini, B. G.; et al. Is buprenorphine transdermal patch equally safe and effective in younger and elderly patients with osteoarthritis-related pain? Results of an age-group controlled study. *Curr. Med. Res. Opin.,* 2013, Dec 23. [Epub ahead of print]

[114] Fareed, A.; Patil, D.; Scheinberg, K.; et al. Comparison of QTc interval prolongation for patients in methadone versus buprenorphine maintenance treatment: a 5-year follow-up. *J. Addict Dis.*, 2013, 32(3), 244-51.

[115] Stallvik, M.; Nordstrand, B.; Kristensen, Ø.; et al. Corrected QT interval during treatment with methadone and buprenorphine – relation to doses and serum concentrations. *Drug Alcohol Depend.*, 2013, 129 (1-2), 88-93.

[116] Jones, H. E.; Heil, S. H.; Baewert, A.; et al. Buprenorphine treatment of opioid-dependent pregnant women: a comprehensive review. *Addiction,* 2012, 107 Suppl. 1, 5-27.

[117] Lindemalm, S.; Nydert, P.; Svensson, J. O.; et al. Transfer of buprenorphine into breast milk and calculation of infant drug dose. *J. Hum. Lact.*, 2009, 25(2), 199-205.

[118] Johnson, R. E.; Jones, H. E.; Jasinksi, D. R.; et al. Buprenorphine treatment of pregnant opioid-dependent women: maternal and neonatal outcomes. *Drug Alcohol Depend.*, 2001, 63, 97-103.

[119] Ilett, K. F.; Hackett, L. P.; Gower, S.; et al. Estimated dose exposure of the neonate to buprenorphine and its metabolite norbuprenorphine via breastmilk during maternal buprenorphine substitution treatment. *Breastfeed Med.*, 2012, 7(4), 269-74.

[120] D'Apolito, K. Breastfeeding and substance abuse. *Clin. Obstet. Gynecol.*, 2013, 56(1), 202-11.

[121] Gower, S; Bartu, A; Ilett, KF; et al. The wellbeing of infants exposed to buprenorphine via breast milk at 4 weeks of age. J Hum Lact, 2014, 1-7, epub ahead of print.

[122] Mello, N. K.; Mendelson, J. H. Buprenorphine suppresses heroin use by heroin addicts. *Science,* 1980, 207, 657–9.

[123] Tompkins, D. A.; Smith, M. T.; Mintzer, M. Z.; et al. A double blind, within subject comparison of spontaneous opioid withdrawal from buprenorphine versus morphine. *J. Pharmacol. Exp. Ther.,* 2014, 348(2), 217-26.

[124] Dum, J.; Bläsig, J.; Herz, A. Buprenorphine: demonstration of physical dependence liability. *Eur. J. Pharmacol.*, 1981, 70, 293–300.

[125] Correia, C. J.; Walsh, S. L.; Bigelow, G. E.; et al. Effects associated with double-blind omission of buprenorphine/naloxone over a 98-h period. *Psychopharmacology*, 2006, 189, 297–306.

[126] Westermeyer, J.; McCance-Katz, E. F. Course and treatment of buprenorphine/naloxone withdrawal: an analysis of case reports. *Am. J. Addict*, 2012, 21, 401–3.

[127] Yanagita, T.; Katoh, S.; Wakasa, V.; et al. Dependence potential of buprenorphine studied in rhesus monkeys. *NIDA Res. Monogr.*, 1982, 41, 208–14.

[128] Buprenorphine-containing Transmucosal products for Opioid Dependence (BTOD) [online]. 2014 [2014 March 2]. Available from: https://www.btodrems.com/SitePages/Welcome.aspx

[129] Hayes, B. D.; Klein-Schwartz, W.; Doyon, S. Toxicity of buprenorphine overdoses in children. *Pediatrics*, 2008, 121, e782-6.

[130] Lovegrove, M.; Hampton, L. M.; Budnitz, D. S. Emergency department visits and hospitalizations for buprenorphine ingestion by children – United States, 2010-2011. *MMWR Morb. Mortal Wkly Rep.,* 2013, 62 (3), 56.

[131] Lavonas, E. J.; Banner, W.; Bradt, P.; et al. Root causes, clinical effects, and outcomes of unintentional exposures to buprenorphine by young children. *J. Pediatr.*, 2013, 163, 1377-83.

[132] Kim, H. K.; Smiddy, M.; Hoffman, R. S.; et al. Buprenorphine may not be as safe as you think: a pediatric fatality from unintentional exposure. *Pediatrics,* 2012, 130(6), e1700-3.

[133] Mégarbane, B.; Buisine, A.; Jacobs F.; et al. Prospective comparative assessment of buprenorphine overdose with heroin and methadone: clinical characteristics and response to antidotal treatment. *J. Subst. Abuse Treat.,* 2010, 38(4), 403-7.

[134] Gal, T. J. Naloxone reversal of buprenorphine-induced respiratory depression. *Clin. Pharmacol. Ther.*, 1989, 45(1), 66-71.

[135] Pirnay, S.; Borron, S. W.; Giudicelli, C. P.; et al. A critical review of the causes of death among post-mortem toxicological investigations: analysis of 34 buprenorphine-associated and 35 methadone-associated deaths. *Addiction*, 2004, 99, 978–88.

[136] Pirnay, S.; Mégarbane, B.; Declèves, X.; et al. Buprenorphine alters desmethylflunitrazepam disposition and flunitrazepam toxicity in rats. *Toxicol. Sci.,* 2008, 106(1), 64-73.

[137] Chang, Y.; Moody, D. E. Effect of benzodiazepines on the metabolism of buprenorphine in human liver microsomes. *Eur. J. Clin. Pharmacol.,* 2005, 60, 875–81.

[138] Kilicarslan, T.; Sellers, E. M. Lack of interaction of buprenorphine with flunitrazepam metabolism. *Am. J. Psychiatry*, 2000, 157, 1164–6.

[139] Gueye, P. N.; Borron, S. W.; Risède, P.; et al. Buprenorphine and midazolam act in combination to depress respiration in rats, *Toxicol. Sci.*, 2002, 65, 107–14.

[140] Pirnay, S. O.; Mégarbane, B.; Borron, S. W.; et al. Effects of various combinations of benzodiazepines with buprenorphine on arterial blood gases in rats. *Basic Clin. Pharmacol. Toxicol.*, 2008, 103, 228–39.

[141] Nielsen, S.; Taylor, D. A. The effect of buprenorphine and benzodiazepines on respiration in the rat. *Drug Alcohol Depend.*, 2005, 79(1), 95–101.

[142] Häkkinen, M.; Launiainen, T.; Vuori, E.; et al. Benzodiazepines and alcohol are associated with cases of fatal buprenorphine poisoning. *Eur. J. Clin. Pharmacol.*, 2012, 68, 301–9.

[143] Lintzeris, N.; Mitchell, T. B.; Bond, A.; et al. Interactions on mixing diazepam with methadone or buprenorphine in maintenance patients. *J. Clin. Psychopharmacol.,* 2006, 26(3), 274-83.

[144] Tracqui, A.; Kintz, P.; Ludes, B. Buprenorphine-related deaths among drug addicts in France: a report on 20 fatalities. *J. Anal. Toxicol.*, 1998, 22(6), 430-4.

[145] Reynaud, M.; Petit, G.; Potard, D.; et al. Six deaths linked to concomitant use of buprenorphine and benzodiazepines. *Addiction,* 1998, 93(9), 1385–92.

[146] Kintz, P. A new series of 13 buprenorphine-related deaths. *Clin. Biochem.*, 2002, 35(7), 513-6.

[147] Lai, S. H.; Yao, Y. J.; Lo, D. S. T. A survey of buprenorphine related deaths in Singapore. *Forensic Sci. Int.*, 2006, 162, 80-6.

[148] Gaulier, J. M.; Marquet, P.; Lacassie, E.; et al. Fatal intoxication following self-administration of a massive dose of buprenorphine. *J. Forensic Sci.*, 2000, 45(1), 226–8.

[149] Papworth, D. P. High dose buprenorphine for postoperative analgesia. *Anesthesia,* 1983, 38(2), 163.

[150] Forrest, A. L. Buprenorphine and lorazepam. *Anaesthesia*, 1983, 38(6), 598.

[151] Maxwell, J. C.; McCance-Katz, E. F. Indicators of buprenorphine and methadone use and abuse: what do we know? *Am. J. Addict*, 2010, 19(1), 73-88.

[152] Schuman-Olivier, Z.; Hoeppner, B. B.; Weiss, R. D.; et al. Benzodiazepine use during buprenorphine treatment for opioid

dependence: clinical and safety outcomes. *Drug Alcohol Depend.*, 2013, 132(3), 580-6.

[153] Guo, A. Y.; Ma, J. D.; Best, B. M.; et al. Urine specimen detection of concurrent nonprescribed medicinal and illicit drug use in patients prescribed buprenorphine. *J. Anal. Toxicol.*, 2013, 37, 636-41.

[154] Otto, M. W.; Bruce, S. E.; Deckersbach, T. Benzodiazepine use, cognitive impairment, and cognitive-behavioral therapy for anxiety disorders: issues in the treatment of a patient in need. *J. Clin. Psychiatry,* 2005, 66 (Suppl 2), 34–8.

[155] Soyka, M. To substitute or not substitute-optimal tactics for the management of benzodiazepine dependence. *Addiction,* 2010, 105, 1876–7.

[156] Brands, B.; Blake, J.; Marsh, D. C.; et al. The impact of buprenorphine use on methadone maintenance treatment outcomes. *J. Addict Dis.,* 2008, 27(3), 37-48.

[157] Bleich, A.; Gelkopf, M.; Schmidt, V.; et al. Correlates of benzodiazepine abuse in methadone maintenance treatment. A 1 year prospective study in an Israeli clinic. *Addiction*, 1999, 94(10), 1533-40.

[158] Brunette, M. F.; Noordsy, D. L.; Xie, H.; et al. Benzodiazepine use and abuse among patients with severe mental illness and co-occurring substance use disorders. *Psychiatr. Serv.*, 2003, 54(10), 1395–1401.

[159] Chen, K. W.; Berger, C. C.; Forde, D. P.; et al. Benzodiazepine use and misuse among patients in a methadone program. *BMC Psychiatry,* 2011, 11(90), 1-7.

[160] Liebrenz, M.; Boesch, L.; Stohler, R.; et al. Agonist substitution—a treatment alternative for high-dose benzodiazepine-dependent patients? *Addiction,* 2010, 105, 1870–4.

[161] Kapil, R. P.; Cipriano, A.; Michels, G. H.; et al. Effect of ketoconazole on the pharmacokinetic profile of buprenorphine following administration of a once-weekly buprenorphine transdermal system. *Clin. Drug Investig.*, 2012, 32(9), 583-92.

[162] Substance Abuse and Mental Health Services Administration, Results from the 2012 National Survey on Drug Use and Health: Summary of National Findings, NSDUH Series H-46, HHS Publication No. (SMA) 13-4795. Rockville, MD: Substance Abuse and Mental Health Services Administration, 2013.

[163] Centers for Disease Control and Prevention (CDC). CDC grand rounds: prescription drug overdoses – a U.S. epidemic. *MMWR Morb. Mortal Wkly Rep.*, 2012, 61(1), 10-3.

[164] Birnbaum, H. G.; White, A. G.; Schiller, M.; et al. Societal costs of prescription opioid abuse, dependence, and misuse in the United States. *Pain Med.,* 2011, 12, 657–67.

[165] Crist, R. C.; Clarke, T. K.; Ang, A.; et al. An intronic variant in OPRD1 predicts treatment outcome for opioid dependence in African-americans. *Neuropsychopharmacology*, 2013, 38(10), 2003-10.

[166] Andrews, C. M.; D'Aunno, T. A.; Pollack, H. A., et al. Adoption of evidence-based clinical innovations: the case of buprenorphine use by opioid treatment programs. *Med. Care Res. Rev*., 2014, 71(1), 43-60.

[167] Bickel, W. K.; Stitzer, M. L.; Bigelow, G. E.; et al. A clinical trial of buprenorphine: Comparison with methadone in the detoxification of heroin addicts. *Clin. Pharmacol. Ther.,* 1988, 43, 72–8.

[168] Johnson, R. E.; Jaffe, J. H.; Fudala, P. J. A controlled trial of buprenorphine treatment for opioid dependence. *JAMA,* 1992, 267, 2750-5.

[169] Ling, W.; Wesson, D. R.; Charuvastra, C.; et al. A controlled trial comparing buprenorphine and methadone main tenance in opioid dependence. *Arch. Gen. Psychiatry*, 1996, 53, 401–7.

[170] Tsui, J. I.; Anderson, B. J.; Strong, D. R.; et al. Craving predicts opioid use in opioid-dependent patients initiating buprenorphine treatment: a longitudinal study. *Am. J. Drug Alcohol Abuse*, 2014, Feb. 12. epub ahead of print.

[171] Amato, L.; Davoli, M.; Ferri, M.; et al. Effectiveness of interventions on opiate withdrawal treatment: an overview of systematic reviews. *Drug Alcohol Depend.*, 2004, 73(3), 219-26.

[172] Fiellin, D. A.; Moore, B. A.; Sullivan, L. E.; et al. Long-term treatment with buprenorphine/naloxone in primary care: results at 2–5 years. *Am. J. Addict,* 2008, 17, 116–20.

[173] Wright, N. M. J.; Sheard, L.; Adams, C. E.; et al. Comparison of methadone and buprenorphine for opiate detoxification (LEEDS trial): a randomised controlled trial. *Br. J. Gen. Pract*., 2011, 61(593), e772-80.

[174] Curcio, F.; Franco, T.; Topa, M.; et al. Buprenorphine/naloxone versus methadone in opioid dependence: a longitudinal survey. *Eur. Rev. Med. Pharmacol. Sci.*, 2011, 15(8), 871-4.

[175] Hser, Y. I.; Saxon, A. J.; Huang, D.; et al. Treatment retention among patients randomized to buprenorphine/naloxone compared to methadone in a multi-site trial. *Addiction,* 2013, 109, 79-87.
[176] Johnson, R. E.; Chutuape, M. A.; Strain, E. C.; et al. A comparison of levomethadol acetate, buprenorphine and methadone for opioid dependence. *N. Engl. J. Med.,* 2000, 343, 1290-7.
[177] Pinto, H.; Maskrey, V.; Swift, L.; et al. The SUMMIT trial: a field comparison of buprenorphine versus methadone maintenance treatment. *J. Subst. Abuse Treat.*, 2010, 39(4), 340-52.
[178] Ridge, G.; Gossop, M.; Lintzeris, N.; et al. Factors associated with the prescribing of buprenorphine or methadone for treatment of opiate dependence. *J. Subst. Abuse Treat.*, 2009, 37(1), 95-100.
[179] World Health Organization. Guidelines for the Psychosocially Assisted Pharmacological Treatment of Opioid Dependence. 2009, WHO, Geneva.
[180] Mitchell, S. G.; Gryczynski, J.; Schwartz, R. P.; et al. A randomized trial of intensive outpatient (IOP) vs. standard outpatient (OP) buprenorphine treatment for African Americans. *Drug Alcohol Depend.*, 2013, 128(3), 222-9.
[181] Myers, D. P.; Augustyniak, M.; Molea, J. Buprenorphine for pain management physicians: a dilemma or a therapeutic alternative? *Tech. Reg. Anesth. Pain Manage,* 2005, 9, 216–220.
[182] Mello, N. K.; Mendelson, J. H. Buprenorphine suppresses heroin use by heroin addicts. *Science,* 1980, 207, 657–9.
[183] Kuhlman, J. J.; Levine, B.; Johnson, R. E.; et al. Relationship of plasma buprenorphine and norbuprenorphine to withdrawal symptoms during dose induction, maintenance and withdrawal from sublingual buprenorphine. *Addiction,* 1998, 93(4), 549-559.
[184] Ling, W.; Charuvastra, C.; Collins, J. F.; et al. Buprenorphine maintenance treatment of opioid dependence: a multicenter, randomized clinical trial. *Addiction,* 1998, 93, 475-86.
[185] Balhara, Y. P. S.; Jain, R. A urinalysis-based study of buprenorphine and non-prescription opioid use among patients on buprenorphine maintenance. *J. Pharmacol. Pharmacother.*, 2012, 3(1), 15-9.
[186] Kosten, T. R.; Kleber, H. D. Buprenorphine detoxification from opioid dependence: a pilot study. *Life Sci.*, 1988, 42(6), 635-41.

[187] Johnson, R. E.; Eissenberg, T.; Stitzer, M. L.; et al. Buprenorphine treatment of opioid dependence: clinical trial of daily versus alternate-day dosing. *Drug Alcohol Depend.*, 1995, 40, 27-35.

[188] Amass, L.; Bickel, W. K.; Higgins, S. T.; et al. A preliminary investigation of outcome following gradual or rapid buprenorphine detoxification. *J. Addict Dis.*, 1995, 13(3), 33-45.

[189] Bickel, W. K.; Amass, L.; Crean, J. P.; et al. Buprenorphine dosing every 1, 2, or 3 days in opioid-dependent patients. *Psychopharmacology,* 1999, 146, 111-8.

[190] Amass, L.; Kamien, J. B.; Mikulich, S. K. Thrice-weekly supervised dosing with the combination buprenorphine-naloxone tablet is preferred to daily supervised dosing by opioid-dependent humans. *Drug Alcohol Depend.*, 2001, 61, 173–81.

[191] Notley, C.; Holland, R.; Maskrey, V.; et al. Regaining control: the patient experience of supervised compared with unsupervised consumption in opiate substitution treatment. *Drug Alcohol Rev.*, 2014, 33(1), 64-70.

[192] Mattick, R. P.; Breen, C.; Kimber, J.; et al. Buprenorphine maintenance versus placebo or methadone maintenance for opioid dependence. *Cochrane Database Syst. Rev.*, 2014, Feb 6, 2, CD0022007.

[193] Heikman, P. K.; Ojanperä, I. A. Inadequate dose of opioid-agonist medication is related to misuse of benzodiazepines. *Addict Disord. Their. Treat.,* 2009, 8, 45-153.

[194] Dunn, K. E.; Sigmon, S. C.; Strain, E. C.; et al. The association between outpatient buprenorphine detoxification duration and clinical treatment outcomes: a review. *Drug Alcohol Depend.*, 2011, 119(1-2), 1-9.

[195] Daniels, A. M.; Salisbury-Afshar, E.; Hoffberg, A.; et al. A novel community-based buprenorphine program: client description and initial outcomes. *J. Addict Med.*, 2014, 8(1), 40-6.

[196] Fiellin, D. A.; O'Connor, P. G.; Chawarski, M.; et al. Methadone maintenance in primary care: a randomized controlled trial. *JAMA,* 2001, 286(14), 1724–31.

[197] Pani, P. P.; Maremmani, I.; Pirastu, R.; et al. Buprenorphine: a controlled clinical trial in the treatment of opioid dependence. *Drug Alcohol Depend.,* 2000, 60, 39–50.

[198] Strain, E. C.; Bigelow, G. E.; Liebson, I. A.; et al. Moderate- vs high-dose methadone in the treatment of opioid dependence: a randomized trial. *JAMA*, 1999, 281(11), 1000–5.

[199] Fiellin, D. A.; Pantalon, M. V.; Chawarski, M. C.; et al. Counseling plus buprenorphine–naloxone maintenance therapy for opioid dependence. *N. Engl. J. Med.*, 2006, 355, 365–74.

[200] Böttcher, M.; Beck, O. Evaluation of buprenorphine CEDIA assay versus GC–MS and ELISA using urine samples from patients in substitution treatment. *J. Anal. Toxicol.,* 2005, 29, 769–76.

[201] Brewer, D. D.; Catalano, R. F.; Haggerty, K.; et al. A meta-analysis of predictors of continued drug use during and after treatment for opiate addiction. *Addiction,* 1998, 93, 73–92.

[202] Ferri, M.; Reid Finlayson, A. J.; Wang L.; et al. Predictive factors for relapse in patients on buprenorphine maintenance. *Am. J. Addict*, 2014, 23(1), 62-7.

[203] Bounes, V.; Palmaro, A.; Lapeyre-Mestre, M.; et al. Long-term consequences of acute pain for patients under methadone or buprenorphine maintenance treatment. *Pain Physician*, 2013, 16(6), E739-47.

[204] Moore, B. A.; Fiellin, D. A.; Barry, D. T.; et al. Primary care office-based buprenorphine treatment: comparison of heroin and prescription opioid dependent patients. *J. Gen. Intern. Med.*, 2007, 22(4), 527-30.

[205] Weiss, R. D.; Potter, J. S.; Fiellin, D. A.; et al. Adjunctive counseling during brief and extended buprenorphine-naloxone treatment for prescription opioid dependence: a 2-phase randomized controlled trial. *Arch. Gen. Psychiatry*, 2011, 68(12), 1238-46.

[206] Segest, E.; Mygind, O.; Bay, H. The influence of prolonged stable methadone maintenance treatment on mortality and employment: an 8-year follow-up. *International J. Addict*, 1990, 25(1), 53-63.

[207] Strain, E. C.; Stitzer, M. L.; Liebson, I. A.; et al. Buprenorphine versus methadone in the treatment of opioid dependence: self-reports, urinalysis, and addiction severity index. *J. Clin. Psychopharmacol.*, 1996, 16(1), 58–67.

[208] Hubbard R. L., French M. T. New perspectives on the benefit-cost and cost-effectiveness of drug abuse treatment. *NIDA Res. Monogr.*, 1991, 113, 94-113.

[209] Tkacz, J.; Volpicelli, J.; Un, H.; et al. Relationship between buprenorphine adherence and health service utilization and costs among opioid dependent patients. *J. Subst. Abuse Treat.*, 2013, epub ahead of print.

[210] Jungen, H.; Andresen-Streichert, H.; Muller, A.; et al. Disaccharides in urine samples as markers of intravenous abuse of methadone and buprenorphine. *J. Anal. Toxicol.*, 2013, 37(9), 652-8.

[211] Auriacombe, M.; Fatséas, M.; Dubernet, J.; et al. French field experience with buprenorphine. *Am. J. Addict*, 2004, 13(Suppl. 1), S17–28.

[212] Emmanuelli, J.; Desenclos, J. C. Harm reduction interventions, behaviours and associated health outcomes in France, 1996–2003. *Addiction,* 2005, 100(11), 1690–700.

[213] Ling, W.; Hillhouse, M.; Domier, C.; et al. Buprenorphine tapering schedule and illicit opioid use. *Addiction,* 2009, 104(2), 256-65.

[214] Murphy, S.; Fishman, P. A.; McPherson, S.; et al. Determinants of buprenorphine treatment for opioid dependence. *J. Subst. Abuse Treat.,* 2014, 46(3), 315-9.

[215] Fischer, G.; Johnson, R. E.; Eder, H.; et al. Treatment of opioid-dependent pregnant women with buprenorphine. *Addiction,* 2000, 95(2), 239-44.

[216] Johnson, R. E.; Jones, H. E.; Fischer, G. Use of buprenorphine in pregnancy: patient management and effects on the neonate. *Drug Alcohol Depend.*, 2003, 70(2 Suppl.), S87-101.

[217] Lacroix, I.; Berrebi, A.; Chaumerliac, C.; et al. Buprenorphine in pregnant opioid-dependent women: first results of a prospective study. *Addiction,* 2004, 99(2), 209-14.

[218] Lejeune, C.; Simmat-Durand, L.; Gourarier L.; et al. Prospective multicenter observational study of 260 infants born to 259 opiate-dependent mothers on methadone or high-dose buprenorphine substitution. *Drug Alcohol Depend.*, 2006, 82(3), 250-7.

[219] Kahila, H.; Saisto, T.; Kivitie-Kallio, S.; et al. A prospective study on buprenorphine use during pregnancy: effects on maternal and neonatal outcome. *Acta Obstet. Gynecol. Scand.*, 2007, 86, 185–90.

[220] Debelak, K.; Morrone, W. R.; O'Grady, K. E.; et al. Buprenorphine + naloxone in the treatment of opioid dependence during pregnancy-initial patient care and outcome data. *Am. J. Addict*, 2013, 22(3), 252-4.

[221] Winklbaur-Hausknost, B.; Jaqsch, R.; Graf-Rohrmeister, K.; et al. Lessons learned from a comparison of evidence-based research in pregnant opioid-dependent women. *Hum. Psychopharmacol. Clin. Exp.,* 2013, 28(1), 15-24.

[222] Heikman, P.; Häkkinen, M.; Gergov, M., et al. Urine naloxone concentration at different phases of buprenorphine maintenance treatment. *Drug Test Anal.*, 2013, Mar. 19, epub ahead of print.

[223] Morgan, D. Drug disposition in mother and foetus. *Clin. Exp. Pharmacol. Physiol.*, 1997, 24, 869-73.

[224] Loebstein, R.; Lalkin, A.; Koren, G. Pharmacokinetic changes during pregnancy and their clinical relevance. *Clin. Pharmacokinet.*, 1997, 33(5), 328-43.

[225] Kacinko, S. L.; Jones, H. E.; Johnson, R. E.; et al. Urinary excretion of buprenorphine, norbuprenorphine, buprenorphine-glucuronide, and norbuprenorphine-glucuronide in pregnant women receiving buprenorphine maintenance treatment. *Clin. Chem.*, 2009, 55, 1177-87.

[226] Anderson, G. D. Pregnancy-induced changes in pharmacokinetics: a mechanistic-based approach. *Clin. Pharmacokinet.*, 2005, 44(10), 989-1008.

[227] Schindler, S. D.; Eder, H.; Ortner, R. et al. Neonatal outcome following buprenorphine maintenance during conception and throughout pregnancy. *Addiction*, 2003, 98(1), 103-10.

[228] Nanovskaya, T.; Deshmukh, S.; Brooks, M.; et al. Transplacental transfer and metabolism of buprenorphine. *J. Pharmacol. Exp. Ther.,* 2002, 300(1), 26-33.

[229] Zharikova, O. L.; Deshmukh, S. J.; Nanovskaya, T. N.; et al. The effect of methadone and buprenorphine on human placental aromatase. *Biochem. Pharmacol.*, 2006, 71(8), 1255-64.

[230] Zharikova, O. L.; Deshmukh, S. J.; Kumar, M.; et al. The effect of opiates on the activity of human placental aromatase/CYP19. *Biochem. Pharmacol.,* 2007, 73(2), 279-86.

[231] O'Connor, A.; Alto, W.; Musgrave, K.; et al. Observational study of buprenorphine treatment of opioid-dependent pregnant women in a family medicine residency: reports on maternal and infant outcomes. J. *Am. Board Fam. Med.,* 2011, 24(2), 194–201.

[232] Lacroix, I.; Berrebi, A.; Garipuy, D.; et al. Buprenorphine versus methadone in pregnant opioid-dependent women: a prospective multicenter study. *Eur. J. Clin. Pharmacol.*, 2011, 67(10), 1053-9.

[233] Metz, V.; Jaqsch, R.; Ebner, N.; et al. Impact of treatment approach on maternal and neonatal outcome in pregnant opioid-maintained women. *Hum. Psychopharmacol.*, 2011, 26(6), 412-21.

[234] Jones, H. E.; Dengler, E.; Garrison, A.; et al. Neonatal outcomes and their relationship to maternal buprenorphine dose during pregnancy. *Drug Alcohol Depend.*, 2014, 134, 414-7.

[235] Carrieri, M. P.; Amass, L.; Lucas, G. M.; et al. Buprenorphine use: the international experience. *Clin. Infect. Dis.*, 2006, 43, S197–215.

[236] Jones, H. E.; Johnson, R. E.; Jasinski, D. R.; et al. Buprenorphine versus methadone in the treatment of pregnant opioid-dependent patients: effects on the neonatal abstinence syndrome. *Drug Alcohol Depend.*, 2005, 79, 1–10.

[237] Kakko, J.; Heilig, M.; Sarman, I. Buprenorphine and methadone treatment of opiate dependence during pregnancy: comparison of fetal growth and neonatal outcomes in two consecutive case series. *Drug Alcohol Depend.,* 2008, 96, 69–78.

[238] Gaalema, D. E.; Scott, T. L.; Heil, S. H.; et al. Differences in the profile of neonatal abstinence syndrome signs in methadone- versus buprenorphine-exposed neonates. *Addiction,* 2012, 107(Suppl. 1), 53-62.

[239] Fischer, A.; Ortner, R.; Rohrmeister, K.; et al. Methadone versus buprenorphine in pregnant addicts: a double-blind, double-dummy comparison study. *Addiction*, 2006, 101(2), 275-81.

[240] Jones, H. E.; Kaltenbach, K.; Heil, S. H.; et al. Neonatal abstinence syndrome after methadone or buprenorphine exposure. *N. Engl. J. Med.,* 2010, 363(24), 2320-31.

[241] Pritham, U. A.; Paul, J. A.; Hayes, M. J. Opioid dependency in pregnancy and length of stay for neonatal abstinence syndrome. *J. Obstet Gynecol. Neonatal. Nurs.*, 2012, 41(2), 180-90.

[242] Kacinko, S. L.; Jones, H. E.; Johnson, R. E.; et al. Correlations of maternal buprenorphine dose, buprenorphine, and metabolite concentrations in meconium with neonatal outcomes. *Clin. Pharmacol. Ther.,* 2008, 84, 604–12.

[243] Bakstad, B.; Sarfi, M.; Welle-Strand, G. K.; et al. Opioid maintenance treatment during pregnancy: occurrence and severity of neonatal

abstinence syndrome. A national prospective study. *Eur. Addict Res.*, 2009, 15(3), 128-34.

[244] Zacny, J.; Bigelow, G.; Compton, P.; et al. College on Problems of Drug Dependence taskforce on prescription opioid non-medical use and abuse: position statement. *Drug Alcohol Depend.*, 2003, 69(3), 215-32.

[245] Luty, J. Treatment preferences of opiate-dependent patients. *Psychiatr. Bull.,* 2004, 28, 47-50.

[246] Appel, P. W.; Ellison, A. A.; Jansky, H. K.; et al. Barriers to enrollment in drug abuse treatment and suggestions for reducing them. *Am. J. Drug Alcohol Abuse,* 2004, 30(1), 129-53.

[247] Kleber, H. D. Pharmacologic treatments for opioid dependence: detoxification and maintenance options. *Dialogues Clin. Neurosci.,* 2007, 9(4), 455-70.

[248] Gryczynski , J.; Mitchell, S. G.; Jaffe, J. H.; et al. Leaving buprenorphine treatment: patients' reasons for cessation of care. *J. Subst. Abuse Treat.*, 2014, 46(3), 356-61.

[249] Cicero, T. J.; Surratt, H.; Inciardi, J. A.; et al. Relationship between therapeutic use and abuse of opioid analgesics in rural, suburban, and urban locations in the United States. *Pharmacoepidemiol. Drug Saf.,* 2007, 16(8), 827-40.

[250] Lenardson, J.; Gale, J. A. Distribution of substance abuse treatment facilities across the rural-urban continuum. US Department of Health and Human Services, Federal Office of Rural Health Policy, 2007 [2014 February 20]. Available from: http://muskie.usm.maine.edu/ Publications/rural /wp35b.pdf. 2007.

[251] Rosenblum, A.; Cleland, C. M.; Fong, C.; et al. Distance traveled and cross-state commuting to opioid treatment programs in the United States. *J. Environ. Public Health*, 2011, 2011(948789), 1-10.

[252] Rounsaville, B. J.; Kosten, T. R. Treatment for opioid dependence: quality and access. *JAMA,* 2000, 283(10), 1337-9.

[253] Iguchi, M. Y.; Stitzer, M. L. Predictors of opiate drug abuse during a 90-daymethadone detoxification. *Am. J. Drug Alcohol Abuse*, 1991, 17(3), 279-94.

[254] Franken, I. H. A.; Hendriks, V. M. Predicting outcome of inpatient detoxification of substance abusers. *Psychiatr. Serv.*, 1999, 50(6), 813-7.

[255] Kampman, K. M.; Pettinati, H. M.; Volpicelli, J. R.; et al. Cocaine dependence severity predicts outcome in outpatient detoxification from cocaine and alcohol. *Am. J. Addict*, 2004, 13(1), 74-82.

[256] Sigmon, S. C. Characterizing the emerging population of prescription opioid abusers. *Am. J. Addict*, 2006, 15(3), 208-12.

[257] Rosenblum, A.; Parrino, M.; Schnoll, S. H.; et al. Prescription opioid abuse among enrollees into methadone maintenance treatment. *Drug Alcohol Depend.*, 2007, 90, 64-71.

[258] Gossop, M.; Griffiths, P.; Bradley, B.; et al. Opiate withdrawal symptoms in response to 10-day and 21-day methadone withdrawal programmes. *Br. J. Psychiatry*, 1989, 154, 360-3.

[259] Woody, G. E.; Poole, S. A.; Subramaniam, G.; et al. Extended vs short-term buprenorphine-naloxone for treatment of opioid-addicted youth: a randomized trial. *JAMA,* 2008, 300(17), 2003-11.

[260] Katz, E. C.; Schwartz, R. P.; King, S.; et al. Brief vs. extended buprenorphine detoxification in a community treatment program: engagement and short-term outcomes. *Am. J. Drug Alcohol Abuse,* 2009, 35(2), 63-7.

[261] Nosyk, B.; Sun, H.; Evans, E.; et al. Defining dosing pattern characteristics of successful tapers following methadone maintenance treatment: results from a population-based retrospective cohort study. *Addiction*, 2012, 107(9), 1621-9.

[262] Sigmon, S. C.; Dunn, K. E.; Saulsgiver, K.; et al. A randomized, double-blind evaluation of buprenorphine taper duration in primary prescription opioid abusers. *JAMA Psychiatry*, 2013. 70(12), 1347-51.

[263] Sanders, N. C.; Mancino, M. J., Gentry, W. B.; et al. Randomized, placebo-controlled pilot trial of gabapentin during an outpatient, buprenorphine-assisted detoxification procedure. *Exp. Clin. Psychopharmacol.*, 2013, 21(4), 294-302.

[264] Becker, A. B.; Strain, E. C.; Bigelow, G. E.; et al. Gradual dose taper following chronic buprenorphine. *Am. J. Addict*, 2001, 10(2), 111–21.

[265] Kornør, H.; Waal, H.; Sandvik, L. Time-limited buprenorphine replacement therapy for opioid dependence: 2-year follow-up outcomes in relation to programme completion and current agonist therapy status. *Drug Alcohol Rev*., 2007, 26, 135-41.

[266] Collins, G. B.; McAllister, M. S. Buprenorphine maintenance: a new treatment for opioid dependence. *Cleve. Clin. J. Med.,* 2007, 74(7), 514–20.

[267] Feng, S.; ElSohly, M. A.; Duckworth, D. T. Hydrolysis of conjugated metabolites of buprenorphine. I. The quantitative enzymatic hydrolysis of buprenorphine-3-beta-D-glucuronide in human urine. *J. Anal. Toxicol.*, 2001, 25, 589-93.

[268] Wallenstein, S. L.; Kaiko, R. F.; Rogers, A. G.; et al. Crossover trials in clinical analgesic assays: Studies of buprenorphine and morphine. *Pharmacotherapy*, 1986, 6(5), 228–35.

[269] Inturrisi, C. E. Clinical pharmacology of opioids for pain. *Clin. J. Pain,* 2002, 18, S3–13.

[270] Lundorff, L.; Sjøgren, P.; Hansen, O. B.; et al. Switching from high doses of pure μ-opioid agonists to transdermal buprenorphine in patients with cancer: a feasibility study. *J. Opioid Manag.*, 2013, 9(4), 255-62.

[271] Miller, K.; Yarlas, A.; Wen, W.; et al. The impact of buprenorphine transdermal delivery system on activities of daily living among patients with chronic low back pain: an application of the international classification of functioning, disability and health. *Clin. J. Pain*, 2014, epub ahead of print.

[272] Samal, S.; Rani, P.; Chandrasekar L. J., et al. Intrathecal buprenorphine or intrathecal dexmedetomidine for postoperative analgesia: a comparative study. *Health Agenda*, 2014, 2(1), 9-14.

[273] Carl, P.; Crawford, M. E.; Madsen, N. B. B.; et al. Pain relief after major abdominal surgery: a double-blind controlled comparison of sublingual buprenorphine, intramuscular buprenorphine, and intramuscular Meperidine. *Anesth. Analg.*, 1987, 66, 142-6.

[274] Payandemehr, P.; Jalili, M.; Davani, B. M.; et al. Sublingual buprenorphine for acute renal colic pain management: a double-blind, randomized controlled trial. *Int. J. Emerg. Med.*, 2014, 7(1).

[275] Bryson, E. O. The perioperative management of patients maintained on medications used to manage opioid addiction. *Curr. Opin. Anaesthesiol.*, 2014, 27, epub ahead of print.

[276] Substance Abuse and Mental Health Services Administration, Center for Behavioral Health Statistics and Quality. (January 29, 2013). The DAWN Report: Emergency Department Visits Involving Buprenorphine. Rockville, MD.

[277] Thomas, K. C.; Malheiro, M.; Crouch, B. I.; et al. Buprenorphine prescribing practices and exposures reported to a poison center – Utah, 2002-2011. *MMWR Morb. Mortal Wkly Rep.*, 2012, 61(49), 997-1001.

[278] European Monitoring Centre for Drugs and Drug Addiction. The state of the drugs problem in Europe: annual report 2012 [online].2012 [2014 February 14]. Available from: http://www.emcdda.europa.eu/publications/annual-report/2012.

[279] Johanson, C. E.; Arfken, C. L.; di Menza, S.; et al. Diversion and abuse of buprenorphine: findings from national surveys of treatment patients and physicians. *Drug Alcohol Depend.*, 2012, 120, 190-5.

[280] Bartholow, M. Top 200 drugs of 2009. *Pharm. Times*, May 2010.

[281] Bartholow, M. Top 200 drugs of 2010. *Pharm. Times,* May 2011.

[282] Bartholow, M. Top 200 drugs of 2011. *Pharm. Times*, July 2012.

[283] Bartholow, M. Top 200 drugs of 2012. *Pharm. Times*, July 2013.

[284] Mello, N. K.; Bree, M. P.; Mendelson, J. H. Buprenorphine self-administration by rhesus monkey. *Pharmacol. Biochem. Behav.*, 1981, 15, 215–25.

[285] Preston, K. L.; Liebson, I. A.; Bigelow, G. E. Discrimination of agonist-antagonist opioids in humans trained on a two-choice saline-hydromorphone discrimination. *J. Pharmacol. Exp. Ther.*, 1992, 261, 62–71.

[286] Preston, K. L.; Bigelow, G. E.; Bickel, W. K.; et al. Drug discrimination in human postaddicts: agonist-antagonist opioids. *J. Pharmacol. Exp. Ther.*, 1989, 250(1), 184–96.

[287] Alho, H.; Sinclair, D.; Vuori, E.; et al. Abuse liability of buprenorphine-naloxone tablets in untreated IV drug users. *Drug Alcohol Depend.*, 2007, 88, 75–8.

[288] Hakansson, A.; Medvedeo, A.; Andersson, M.; et al. Buprenorphine misuse among heroin and amphetamine users in Malmo, Sweden: purpose of misuse and route of administration. *Eur. Addict Res.,* 2007, 13(4), 207–15.

[289] Schuman-Olivier, Z.; Albanese, M.; Nelson, S. E.; et al. Self-treatment: illicit buprenorphine use by opioid-dependent treatment seekers. *J. Subst. Abuse Treat.*, 2010, 39(1), 41–50.

[290] Larance, B.; Lintzeris, N.; Ali, R.; et al. The diversion and injection of a buprenorphine-naloxone soluble film formulation. *Drug Alcohol Depend.*, 2014, 136, 21-7.

[291] Bazazi, A.R.; Yokell, M.; Fu, J. J.; et al. Illicit use of buprenorphine/naloxone among injecting and non-injecting opioid users. *J. Add. Med.*, 2011, 5, 175-80.

[292] National Drug Intelligence Center. Heroin: National Drug Threat Assessment 2003 [online]. January 2003 [2014 March 5]. Available from: http://www.justice.gov/archive/ndic/pubs3/3300/heroin.htm

[293] Kumar, M.; Mudaliar, S.; Thyagarajan, S.; et al. Rapid assessment and response to injecting drug use in Madras, south India. *Int. J. Drug Policy,* 2000, 11(1–2), 83– 98.

[294] Aitken, C. K.; Higgs, P. G.; Hellard, M. E. Buprenorphine injection in Melbourne, Australia – an update. *Drug Alcohol Rev.*, 2008, 27, 197–9.

[295] O'Connor, J. J.; Moloney, E.; Travers, R.; et al. Buprenorphine abuse among opiate addicts. *Br. J. Addict,* 1988, 83, 1085–7.

[296] Sakol, M. S.; Stark, C.; Sykes, R. Buprenorphine and temazepam abuse by drug takers in Glasgow—an increase. *Brit. J. Addict.,* 1989, 84, 439–41.

[297] Lavelle, T. L.; Hammersley, R.; Forsyth, A. The use of buprenorphine and temazepam by drug injectors. *J. Addict Dis.*, 1991, 10(3), 5–14.

[298] Kintz, P.; Villain, M.; Tracqui, A.; et al. Buprenorphine in drug-facilitated sexual abuse: a fatal case involving a 14-year-old boy. *J. Anal. Toxicol.,* 2003, 27(7), 527-9.

[299] Harper, I. Temgesic abuse [letter]. *NZ Med. J.,* 1983, 96, 777.

[300] Strang, J. Abuse of buprenorphine. *Lancet,* 1985, 2(8457), 725.

[301] Robinson, G. M.; Dukes, P. D.; Robinson, B. J.; et al. The misuse of buprenorphine and a buprenorphine-naloxone combination in Wellington, New Zealand. *Drug Alcohol Depend.*, 1993, 33, 81–6.

[302] Chai, L. Y. A.; Khare, C. B.; Chua, A.; et al. Buprenorphine diversion: a possible reason for increased incidence of infective endocarditis among injection drug users? The Singapore experience. *Clin. Infect. Dis.,* 2008, 46, 953–5.

[303] Solomon, S. S.; Desai, M.; Srikrishnan, A.; et al. The profile of injection drug users in Chennai, India: identification of risk behaviours and implications for interventions. *Subst. Use Misuse*, 2010, 45(3), 354-67.

[304] Cassidy, T. A.; DasMahapatra, P.; Black, R. A.; et al. Changes in prevalence of prescription opioid abuse after introduction of an abuse-deterrent opioid formulation. *Pain Med.*, 2013, Dec 11. doi: 10.1111/pme.12295.

[305] Substance Abuse and Mental Health Services Administration. Drug Abuse Warning Network (DAWN), National Estimates of Drug-Related Emergency Department Visits, 2004 – 2011.

[306] CESAR FAX. Fentanyl and buprenorphine have higher rates of nonmedical use ED visits per dosage units distributed to retail outlets than other opioids. CESAR FAX; 2011;20(28).

[307] Wish, E. D.; Artigiani, E.; Billing, A.; et al. The emerging buprenorphine epidemic in the United States. *J. Addict Dis.*, 2012, 31(1), 3-7.

[308] CESAR FAX. Thus far in 2012 more than one-half of U.S. states have had media reports of buprenorphine misuse or diversion. CESAR FAX 2012;21(38).

[309] Kintz, P. Deaths involving buprenorphine: a compendium of cases. *Forensic Sci. Int.*, 2001, 121, 65-9.

[310] U.S. Drug Enforcement Administration, Office of Diversion Control. National Forensic Laboratory Information System: year 2012 annual report. 2013, Springfield, VA: U.S. Drug Enforcement Administration.

[311] Feroni, I.; Peretti-Watel, P.; Paraponaris, A.; et al. French general practitioners' attitudes and prescription patterns toward buprenorphine maintenance treatment: does doctor shopping reflect buprenorphine misuse? *J. Addict Dis.,* 2005, 24(3), 7-22.

[312] Nielsen, S.; Dietze, P.; Dunlop, A.; et al. Buprenorphine supply by community pharmacists in Victoria, Australia: perceptions, experiences, and key issues identified. *Drug Alcohol Rev.*, 2007, 26, 143-51.

[313] Larance, B.; Degenhardt, L.; Lintzeris, N.; et al. Post-marketing surveillance of buprenorphine-naloxone in Australia: diversion, injection and adherence with supervised dosing. *Drug Alcohol Depend.*, 2011, 118(2-3), 265-73.

[314] Winstock, A. R. Buprenorphine use by the smoking route in gaols in NSW. *Drug Alcohol Rev.*, 2008, 27, 449–50.

[315] Jenkinson, R. A.; Clark, N. C.; Fry, C. L.; et al. Buprenorphine diversion and injection in Melbourne, Australia: an emerging issue? *Addiction,* 2005, 100, 197–205.

[316] Wade, L.; Bridgeman, M. B.; Pathak, R. Novel tactics: deterring opioid abuse. Pharm Times [online]. August 16, 2012 [2014 February 14]. Available from: http://www.pharmacytimes.com/publications/issue/2012/August2012/Novel-Tactics-Deterring-Opioid-Abuse#

[317] Hammersley, R.; Lavelle, T.; Forsyth, A. Predicting initiation to and cessation of buprenorphine and temazepam use amongst adolescents. *Br. J. Addict.*, 1992, 87(9), 1303-11.

[318] Uosukainen, H.; Ilomäki, J.; Kauhanen, J.; et al. Factors associated with buprenorphine compared to amphetamine abuse among clients seeking treatment in Finland. *J. Subst. Abuse Treat.*, 2014, doi: 10.1016/j.jsat.2014.01.004

[319] Bruce, R. D.; Govindasamy, S.; Sylla, L.; et al. Lack of reduction in buprenorphine injection after introduction of co-formulated buprenorphine/naloxone to the Malaysian market. *Am. J. Drug Alcohol Abuse,* 2009, 35(2), 68-72.

[320] Vicknasingam, B.; Mazlan, M.; Schottenfeld, R. S.; et al. Injection of buprenorphine and buprenorphine/naloxone tablets in Malaysia. *Drug Alcohol Depend.*, 2010, 111(1-2), 44-9.

[321] Cone, E. J.; Caplan, Y. H.; Black, D. L.; et al. Urine drug testing of chronic pain patients: licit and illicit drug patterns. *J. Anal. Toxicol.*, 2008, 32, 530-43.

[322] Winstock, A. R.; Lea, T. Diversion and injection of methadone and buprenorphine among clients in public opioid treatment clinics in New South Wales, Australia. *Subst. Use Misuse*, 2010, 45(1– 2), 240–52.

[323] Obadia, Y.; Perrin, V.; Feroni, I.; et al. Injecting misuse of buprenorphine among French drug users. *Addiction*, 2001, 96(2), 267–72.

[324] Ferrant, O.; Papin, F.; Clin, B.; et al. Fatal poisoning due to snorting buprenorphine and alcohol consumption. *Forensic Sci. Int.*, 2011, 204(1-3), e8-11.

[325] Horyniak, D.; Dietze, P.; Larance, B.; et al. The prevalence and correlates of buprenorphine inhalation amongst opioid substitution treatment (OST) clients in Australia. *Int. J. Drug Policy*, 2011, 22, 167-71.

[326] Becker, A. B.; Bigelow, G. E.; Liebson, I. A. Transdermal buprenorphine: Abuse potential assessment in non-opioid-dependent volunteers [abstract]. *Drug Alcohol Depend.*, 2001, 63(Suppl 1), S13.

[327] Auriacombe, M.; Franques, P.; Tignol, J. Deaths attributable to methadone vs buprenorphine in France. *JAMA*, 2001, 285(1), 45.

[328] Vincent, F.; Bessard, J.; Vacheron, J.; et al. Determination of buprenorphine and norbuprenorphine in urine and hair by gas chromatography–mass spectrometry. *J. Anal. Toxicol.*, 1999, 23, 270–9.

[329] Häkkinen, M.; Heikman, P.; Ojanperä, I. Parenteral buprenorphine-naloxone abuse is a major cause of fatal buprenorphine-related poisoning. *Forensic Sci. Int.*, 2013, 232(1-3), 11-5.

[330] Druid, H.; Strandberg, J. J.; Alkass, K.; et al. Evaluation of the role of abstinence in heroin overdose deaths using segmental hair analysis. *Forensic Sci. Int.*, 2007, 168, 223–6.

[331] Tagliaro, F.; De Battisti, Z.; Smith, F. P.; et al. Death from heroin overdose: findings from hair analysis, *Lancet,* 1998, 351, 1923–5.

[332] Fugelstad, A.; Ahlner, J.; Brandt, L.; et al. Use of morphine and 6-monoacetylmorphine in blood for the evaluation of possible risk factors for sudden death in 192 heroin users. *Addiction,* 2003, 98, 463–70.

[333] Kronstrand, R.; Nyström, I.; Strandberg, J.; et al. Screening for drugs of abuse in hair with ion spray LC–MS–MS. *Forensic Sci. Int.,* 2004, 145, 183–90.

[334] Kronstrand, R.; Nyström, I.; Andersson, M.; et al. Urinary detection times and metabolite/parent compound ratios after a single dose of buprenorphine. *J. Anal. Toxicol.*, 2008, 32(8), 586-93.

[335] Soyka, M.; Penning, R.; Wittchen, U. Fatal poisoning in methadone and buprenorphine treated patients – are there differences? *Pharmacopsychiatry*, 2006, 39(3), 85–7.

[336] Stanton A., McLeod C., Kissin W.; et al. Evaluation of the Buprenorphine Waiver Program: Results from SAMHSA/CSAT's evaluation of the Buprenorphine Waiver Program. *NIDA Res. Monogr.,* 2006, 186.

[337] Cone, E. J.; Dickerson, S. L. Efficacy of urinanalysis in monitoring heroin and cocaine abuse patterns: implications in clinical trials for treatment of drug dependence. *NIDA Res. Monogr.*, 1992, 128, 46-58.

[338] Pesce, A.; West, C.; City, K. E.; et al. Interpretation of urine drug testing in pain patients. *Pain Medicine*, 2012, 13, 868-85.

[339] Melanson, S. E. F.; Kredlow, M. I.; Jarolim, P. Analysis and interpretation of drug testing results from patients on chronic pain therapy: a clinical laboratory perspective. *Clin. Chem. Lab. Med.,* 2009, 47, 971–6.

[340] Pesce, A.; Gonzales, E.; Almazan, P.; et al. Medication and illicit substance use analyzed using liquid chromatography tandem mass spectrometry (LC-MS/MS) in a pain population. *J. Anal. Bioanal. Techniques*, 2012, 3, 135. doi:10.4172/2155-9872.1000135.

[341] Cone, E. J.; Gorodetzky, C. W.; Yousefnejad, D.; et al. 63Ni electron-capture gas chromatographic assay for buprenorphine and metabolites in human urine and feces. *J. Chromatogr.*, 1985, 337, 291-300.

[342] Hand, C. W.; Ryan, K. E.; Dutt, S. K.; et al. Radioimmunoassay of buprenorphine in urine: studies in patients and in a drug clinic. *J. Anal. Toxicol.*, 1989, 13(2), 100-4.

[343] Debrabandere, L.; Van Boven, M.; Daenens, P. High-performance liquid chromatography with electrochemical detection of buprenorphine and its major metabolite in urine. *J. Chromatogr.*, 1991, 564, 557–66.

[344] Blom, Y.; Bondesson, U.; Anggard, E. Analysis of buprenorphine and its N-dealkylated metabolite in plasma and urine by selected-ion monitoring. *J. Chromatogr.*, 1985, 338, 89–98.

[345] Lisi, A. M.; Kazlauskas, R.; Trout, G. J. Gas chromatographic–mass spectrometric quantitation of urinary buprenorphine and norbuprenorphine after derivatization by direct extractive alkylation. *J. Chromatogr. B. Biomed. Sci. Appl.*, 1997, 692(1), 67–77.

[346] George, S.; George, C.; Chauhan, M. The development and application of a rapid gas chromatography–mass spectrometry method to monitor buprenorphine withdrawal protocols. *Forensic Sci. Int.*, 2004, 143, 121–5.

[347] Strano-Rossi, S.; Bermejo, A. M.; de la Torre, X., et al. Fast GC-MS method for the simultaneous screening of THC-COOH, cocaine, opiates and analogues including buprenorphine and fentanyl, and their metabolites in urine. *Anal. Bioanal. Chem.*, 2011, 399(4), 1623-30.

[348] Kronstrand, R.; Seldén, T. G.; Josefsson, M. Analysis of buprenorphine, norbuprenorphine, and their glucuronides in urine by liquid chromatography–mass spectrometry. *J. Anal. Toxicol.*, 2003, 27, 464–70.

[349] Fox, E. J.; Tetlow, V. A.; Allen, K. R. Quantitative analysis of buprenorphine and norbuprenorphine in urine using liquid chromatography tandem mass spectrometry. *J. Anal. Toxicol.*, 2006, 30, 238–44.

[350] Hegstad, S.; Khiabani H. Z.; Øiestad E. L.; et al. Rapid quantification of buprenorphine-glucuronide and norbuprenorphine-glucuronide in human urine by LC-MS-MS. *J. Anal. Toxicol.*, 2007, 31(4), 214-9.

[351] Huang, W.; Moody, D. E.; McCance-Katz, E. F. The in vivo glucuronidation of buprenorphine and norbuprenorphine determined by liquid chromatography-electrospray ionization-tandem mass spectrometry. *Ther. Drug Monit.*, 2006, 28, 245-51.

[352] McMillin, G. A.; Davis, R.; Carlisle, H.; et al. Patterns of free (unconjugated) buprenorphine, norbuprenorphine, and their glucuronides in urine using liquid chromatography-tandem mass spectrometry. *J. Anal. Toxicol.*, 2012, 36(2), 81-7.

[353] Smith, M. L. Immunoassay. In: Levine B, ed. Principles of Forensic Toxicology. 4th ed. Washington, D.C.: AACC Press; 2013; 149-69.

[354] Standridge, J. B.; Adams, S. M.; Zotos, A. P. Urine drug screening: a valuable office procedure. *Am. Fam. Physician*, 2010, 81(5), 635-40.

[355] Zhang, H.; Gelernter, J.; Gruen, J. R.; et al. Functional impact of a single-nucleotide polymorphism in the OPRD1 promoter region. *J. Hum. Genet.*, 2010, 55(5), 278–84.

[356] Dickerson, J. A.; Laha, T. J.; Pagano M. B.; et al. Improved detection of opioid use in chronic pain patients through monitoring of opioid glucuronides in urine. *J. Anal. Toxicol.*, 2012, 36(8), 541-7.

[357] Melanson, S. E.; Snyder, M. L.; Jarolim, P.; et al. A new highly specific buprenorphine immunoassay for monitoring buprenorphine compliance and abuse. *J. Anal. Toxicol.*, 2012, 36(3), 201-6.

[358] Cirimele, V.; Kintz, P.; Lohner, S.; et al. Enzyme immunoassay validation for the detection of buprenorphine in urine. *J. Anal. Toxicol.*, 2003, 27, 103–5.

[359] Shaikh, S.; Hull, M. J.; Bishop, K. A.; et al. Effect of tramadol use on three point-of-care and one instrument-based immunoassays for urine buprenorphine. *J. Anal. Toxicol.*, 2008, 32, 339–43.

[360] Wu, M. Y.; Wang, Y. S.; Lin, C. C.; et al. An empirical study on the selection of analytes and corresponding cutoffs for immunoassay and GC–MS in a two-step test strategy-buprenorphine example. *Analyst*, 2009, 134, 1848–56.

[361] Miller, E. I.; Torrance, H. J.; Oliver, J. S. Validation of Immunalysis microplate ELISA for the detection of buprenorphine and its metabolite norbuprenorphine in urine. *J. Anal. Toxicol.*, 2006, 30, 115–9.

[362] Alves, M. N. R.; Piccinotti, A.; Tameni, S.; et al. Evaluation of buprenorphine LUCIO immunoassay versus GC-MS using urines from a workplace drug testing program. *J. Anal. Toxicol.*, 2013, 37(3), 175-8.

[363] Wang, G. J.; Vincent, M.; Rodrigues, W.; et al. Development and GC–MS validation of a highly sensitive recombinant G6PDH-based homogenous immunoassay for the detection of buprenorphine and norbuprenorphine in urine. *J. Anal. Toxicol.*, 2007, 31, 377–82.

[364] Pavlic, M.; Libiseller, K.; Grubwieser, P.; et al. Cross-reactivity of the CEDIA buprenorphine assay with opiates: An Austrian phenomenon? *Int. J. Leg. Med.*, 2005, 119, 378–81.

[365] Birch, M. A.; Couchman, L.; Pietromartire, S.; et al. False-positive buprenorphine by CEDIA in patients prescribed amisulpride or sulpiride. *J. Anal. Toxicol.*, 2013, 37(4), 233-6.

[366] Basilicata, P.; Pieri, M.; Settembre, V.; et al. Screening of several drugs of abuse in Italian workplace drug testing: performance comparisons of on-site screening tests and a fluorescence polarization immunoassay-based device. *Anal. Chem.*, 2011, 83(22), 8566-74.

[367] Hull, M. J.; Bierer, M. F.; Griggs, D. A.; et al. Urinary buprenorphine concentrations in patients treated with Suboxone as determined by liquid chromatography–mass spectrometry and CEDIA immunoassay. *J. Anal. Toxicol.*, 2008, 32, 516–21.

[368] DePriest, A.; Heltsley, R.; Black, D. L.; et al. Urine drug testing of chronic pain patients. III. Normetabolites as biomarkers of synthetic opioid use. *J. Anal. Toxicol.*, 2010, 34, 444-9.

[369] Heltsley, R.; DePriest, A.; Black, D. L.; et al. Oral fluid drug testing of chronic pain patients. I. Positive prevalence rates of licit and illicit drugs. *J. Anal. Toxicol.*, 2011, 35, 529-40.

[370] Pesce, A.; West, C.; West, R.; et al. Analytical considerations when monitoring pain medications by LC-MS/MS. *J. Anal. Bioanal. Techniques,* 2012, S5:003. doi.10.4172/2155-9872.S5-003.

[371] Moody, D. E.; Laycock, J. D.; Spanbauer, A. C.; et al. Determination of buprenorphine in human plasma by gas chromatography- positive ion chemical ionization mass spectrometry and liquid chromatography-tandem mass spectrometry. *J. Anal. Toxicol.*, 1997, 21, 406–14.

[372] Hegstad, S.; Hermansson, S.; Betnér, I.; et al. Screening and quantitative determination of drugs of abuse in diluted urine by UPLC-MS/MS. *J.*

Chromatogr. B. Analyt. Technol. Biomed. Life Sci., 2014, 947-948, 83-95.

[373] Lippi, G.; Romero, A.; Cervellin, G.; et al. Unusual false-positive case of urinary screening for buprenorphine. *J. Clin. Lab. Anal.*, 2011, 25(4), 244-5.

[374] Greenwald, M. K.; Johanson, C. E.; Moody, D. E.; et al. Effects of buprenorphine maintenance dose on mu-opioid receptor availability, plasma concentrations, and antagonist blockade in heroin-dependent volunteers. *Neuropsychopharmacology,* 2003, 28, 2000–9.

[375] Chawarski, M. C.; Schottenfeld, R. S.; O'Conner, P. G.; et al. Plasma concentrations of buprenorphine 24 to 72 hours after dosing. *Drug Alcohol Depend.*, 1999, 55(1-2), 157-63.

[376] Wilkins, D. G.; Rollins, D. E.; Valdez, A. S.; et al. A retrospective study of buprenorphine and norbuprenorphine in human hair after multiple doses. *J. Anal. Toxicol.*, 1999, 23(6), 409-15.

[377] De Giovanni, N.; Fucci, N.; Scarlata, S.; et al. Buprenorphine detection in biological samples. *Clin. Chem. Lab. Med.*, 2005, 43(12), 1377-9.

[378] White, J.; Bell, J.; Saunders, J. B.; et al. Open-label dose-finding trial of buprenorphine implants (Probuphine)® for treatment of heroin dependence. *Drug Alcohol Depend.*, 2009, 103(1-2), 37-43.

[379] Bartu, A. E.; Ilett, K. F.; Hackett, L. P.; et al. Buprenorphine exposure in infants of opioid-dependent mothers at birth. *Aust. N. Z. J. Obstet. Gynaecol.,* 2012, 52(4), 342-7.

[380] Concheiro, M.; Jones, H. E., Johnson, R. E.; et al. Preliminary buprenorphine sublingual tablet pharmacokinetic data in plasma, oral fluid, and sweat during treatment of opioid-dependent pregnant women. *Ther. Drug Monit.*, 2011, 33(5), 619-26.

[381] Allen, K. R.. Screening for drugs of abuse: which matrix, oral fluid or urine? *Ann. Clin. Biochem.*, 2011, 48, 531-41.

[382] Al-Asmari, A. I.; Anderson, R. A. Comparison of nonhydrolysis and hydrolysis methods for determination of buprenorphine metabolites in urine by liquid chromatography-tandem mass spectrometry. *J. Anal. Toxicol.*, 2008, 32, 744-53.

[383] ElSohly, M. A.; Gul, W.; Feng, S. X.; et al. Hydrolysis of conjugated metabolites of buprenorphine. II. The quantitative enzymatic hydrolysis of norbuprenorphine-3-beta-D-glucuronide in human urine. *J. Anal. Toxicol.*, 2005, 29, 570-3.

[384] Kacinko, S. L.; Concheiro-Guisan, M.; Shakleya, D. M.; et al. Development and validation of a liquid chromatography-tandem mass spectrometry assay for the simultaneous quantification of buprenorphine, norbuprenorphine, and metabolites in human urine. *Anal. Bioanal. Chem.*, 2008, 392, 903-11.

[385] Vignali, C.; Stramesi, C.; Morini, L.; et al. Workplace drug testing in Italy - critical considerations. *Drug Test Anal.*, 2013, 5(4), 208-12.

[386] Pesce, A.; West, C.; West, R.; et al. Reference intervals: a novel approach to detect drug abuse in a pain patient population. *J. Opioid Manag.*, 2010, 6(5), 341-50.

[387] Pesce, A.; West, C.; West, R.; et al. Determination of medication cutoff values in a pain patient population. *J. Opioid Manag.*, 2011, 7(2), 117-22.

[388] Fishman, J.; Roffwarg, H.; Hellman, L. Disposition of naloxone-7,8-3H in normal and narcotic-dependent men. *J. Pharmacol. Exp. Ther.*, 1973, 187(3), 575–80.

[389] Cone, E. J.; Preston, K. L. Toxicologic aspects of heroin substitution treatment. *Ther. Drug Monit.*, 2002, 24(2), 193-8.

[390] Department of Health and Human Services, Substance Abuse and Mental Health Services Administration. Mandatory Guidelines for Federal Workplace Drug Testing Programs; Notice. *Fed. Regist.*, 2008, 73, 71858.

[391] Fraser, A. D.; Zamecnik, J. Impact of lowering the screening and confirmation cutoff values for urine drug testing based on dilution indicators. *Ther. Drug Monit.*, 2003, 25(6), 723-7.

[392] DePriest, A.; Black, D. L.; Robert, T.; et al. Interpretation of urine specimens containing prescription drugs without metabolites: adulteration, impaired metabolism, or normal excretion? Abstract, Society of Forensic Toxicologists, 2013.

[393] Vindenes, V.; Yttredal, B.; Oiestad, E. L., et al. Oral fluid is a viable alternative for monitoring drug abuse: detection of drugs in oral fluid by liquid chromatography-tandem mass spectrometry and comparison to the results from urine samples from patients treated with Methadone or Buprenorphine. *J. Anal. Toxicol.*, 2011, 35(1), 32-9.

[394] Heltsley, R.; DePriest, A.; Black, D. L.; et al. Oral fluid drug testing of chronic pain patients. II. Comparison of paired oral fluid and urine specimens. *J. Anal. Toxicol.*, 2012, 36, 75-80.

[395] Conermann, T.; Gosalia, A. R.; Kabazie, A. J.; et al. Utility of oral fluid in compliance monitoring of opioid medications. *Pain Physician*, 2014, 17, 63-70.

[396] DePriest, A. Z.; Knight, J. L.; Puet, B. L.; et al. Oral fluid testing. *MRO Alert,* 2012, 23(10), 1-5.

[397] Duxbury, K.; Romagnoli, C.; Anderson, M.; et al. Development of a clinically relevant liquid chromatography tandem mass spectrometry assay for 13 drugs of abuse in urine, designed to meet the needs of the service users. *Ann. Clin. Biochem*., 2010, 47(5), 415-22.

[398] Cone, E. J.; Clarke, J.; Tsanaclis, L. Prevalence and disposition of drugs of abuse and opioid treatment drugs in oral fluid. *J. Anal. Toxicol*., 2007, 31(8), 424-33.

[399] Concheiro, M.; Gray, T. R.; Shakleya, D. M. et al. High-throughput simultaneous analysis of buprenorphine, methadone, cocaine, opiates, nicotine, and metabolites in oral fluid by liquid chromatography tandem mass spectrometry. *Anal. Bioanal. Chem*., 2010, 398(2), 915-24.

[400] Cone, E. J.; Huestis, M. A. Interpretation of oral fluid tests for drugs of abuse. *Ann. N Y Acad. Sci*., 2007, 1098, 51-103.

[401] Cone, E. J.; Dickerson, S. L.; Darwin, W. D.; et al. Elevated drug saliva levels suggest a "depot-like" effect in subjects treated with sublingual buprenorphine. *NIDA Res. Monogr*., 1990, 105, 569.

[402] Hegstad, S.; Khiabani, H. Z.; Kristoffersen, L.; et al. Drug screening of hair by liquid chromatography-tandem mass spectrometry. *J. Anal. Toxicol*., 2008, 32(5), 364-72.

[403] Wilkins, D. G.; Valdez, A. S.; Nagasawa, P. R.; et al. Incorporation of drugs for the treatment of substance abuse into pigmented and nonpigmented hair. *J. Pharm. Sci.,* 1998, 87(4), 435-40.

[404] Kintz, P. Segmental hair analysis can demonstrate external contamination in postmortem cases. *Forensic Sci. Int*., 2012, 215(1-3), 73-6.

[405] Goodwin, R. S.; Wilkins, D. G.; Averin, O.; et al. Buprenorphine and norbuprenorphine in hair of pregnant women and their infants after controlled buprenorphine administration. *Clin. Chem*., 2007, 53(12), 2136-43.

[406] Cirimele, V.; Kintz, P. Lohner, S.; et al. Buprenorphine to norbuprenorphine ratio in human hair. J. Anal. Toxicol., 2000, 24(6), 448-9.

[407] Skopp, G.; Kniest, A.; Haisser, J.; et al. Buprenorphine and norbuprenorphine findings in hair during constant maintenance dosage. *Int. J. Legal Med.*, 2011, 125, 277-81.

[408] Kintz, P. Determination of buprenorphine and its dealkylated metabolite in human hair. *J. Anal. Toxicol.*, 1993, 17(7), 443-4.

[409] Kintz, P.; Cirimele, V.; Edel, Y.; et al. Hair analysis for buprenorphine and its dealkylated metabolite by RIA and confirmation by LC/ECD. *J. Forensic Sci.*, 1994, 39(6), 1497-503.

[410] Tracqui, A.; Kintz, P.; Mangin, P. HPLC/MS determination of buprenorphine and norbuprenorphine in biological fluids and hair samples. *J. Forensic Sci.,* 1997, 42(1), 111-4.

[411] Svaizer, F.; Lotti, A.; Gottardi, M.; et al. Buprenorphine detection in hair samples by immunometric screening test: preliminary experience. *Forensic Sci. Int.,* 2010, 196(1-3), 118-20.

[412] Musshoff, F.; Lachenmeier, K.; Trafkowski, J.; et al. Determination of opioid analgesics in hair samples using liquid chromatography/tandem mass spectrometry and application to patients under palliative care. *Ther. Drug Monit.*, 2007, 29(5), 655-61.

[413] Chawarski, M. C.; Fiellin, D. A.; O'Connor, P. G.; et al. Utility of sweat patch testing for drug use monitoring in outpatient treatment for opiate dependence. *J. Subst. Abuse Treat.*, 2007, 33(4), 411-5.

[414] Lozano, J.; Garcia-Algar, O.; Vall, O.; et al. Biological matrices for the evaluation of in utero exposure to drugs of abuse. *Ther. Drug Monit.,* 2007, 29, 711–34.

[415] Concheiro, M.; Shakleya, D. M.; Huestis, M. A. Simultaneous analysis of buprenorphine, methadone, cocaine, opiates and nicotine metabolites in sweat by liquid chromatography tandem mass spectrometry. *Anal. Bioanal. Chem.*, 2011, 400(1), 69-78.

[416] Kintz, P.; Tracqui, A.; Mangin, P.; et al. Sweat testing in opioid users with a sweat patch. *J. Anal. Toxicol.*, 1996, 20(6), 393-7.

[417] De Giovanni, N.; Fucci, N. The current status of sweat testing for drugs of abuse: a review. *Curr. Med. Chem.*, 2013, 20, 545-61.

[418] Beck, O.; Stephanson, N.; Sandqvist, S.; et al. Detection of drugs of abuse in exhaled breath from users following recovery from intoxication. *J. Anal. Toxicol.*, 2012, 36(9), 638-46.

[419] Beck, O.; Stephanson, N.; Sandgvist, S.; et al. Detection of drugs of abuse in exhaled breath using a device for rapid collection: comparison

with plasma, urine and self-reporting in 47 drug users. *J. Breath Res.*, 2013, 7(2), 1-11.

[420] Beck, O. Exhaled breath for drugs of abuse testing – evaluation in criminal justice settings. *Sci. Justice*, 2014, 54(1), 57-60.

[421] Bullingham, R. E. S.; McQuay, H. J.; Moore, A; et al. Buprenorphine kinetics. *Clin. Pharmacol. Ther.*, 1980, 28, 667–72.

[422] Everhart, E. T.; Cheung, P.; Shwonek, P.; et al. Subnanogram-concentration measurement of buprenorphine in human plasma by electron-capture capillary gas chromatography: application to pharmacokinetics of sublingual buprenorphine. *Clin. Chem.*, 1997, 43, 2292-302.

[423] de los Cabos, J. P.; Martin, S.; Etcheberrigaray, A.; et al. A controlled trial of daily versus thrice-weekly buprenorphine administration for the treatment of opioid dependence. *Drug Alcohol Depend.*, 2000, 59, 223-33.

[424] Lanier, R. K.; Umbricht, A.; Harrison, J. A.; et al. Opioid detoxification via single 7-day application of a buprenorphine transdermal patch: an open-label evaluation. *Psychopharmacology*, 2008, 198, 149-58.

[425] Cirimele, V.; Etienne, S.; Villain, M.; et al. Evaluation of the One-Step™ ELISA kit for the detection of buprenorphine in urine, blood, and hair specimens. *Forensic Sci. Int.*, 2004, 143, 153-6.

[426] Ristimaa, J.; Gergov, M.; Pelander, A.; et al. Broad-spectrum drug screening of meconium by liquid chromatography with tandem mass spectrometry and time-of-flight mass spectrometry. *Anal. Bioanal. Chem.*, 2010, 398(2), 925-35.

[427] Gray, T.; Huestis, M. Bioanalytical procedures for monitoring in utero drug exposure. *Anal. Bioanal. Chem.*, 2007, 388, 1455–65.

[428] Kraft, W. K.; Gibson, E.; Dysart, K.; et al. Sublingual buprenorphine for treatment of neonatal abstinence syndrome: a randomized trial. *Pediatrics*, 2008, 122(3), e601-7.

[429] Hytinantti, T.; Kahila, H.; Renlund, M.; et al. Neonatal outcome of 58 infants exposed to maternal buprenorphine in utero. *Acta. Paediatr.*, 2008, 97, 1040–4.

[430] Kacinko, S. L.; Shakleya, D. M.; Huestis, M. A. Validation and application of a method for the determination of buprenorphine, norbuprenorphine, and their glucuronide conjugates in human meconium. *Anal. Chem.*, 2008, 80, 246–52.

[431] Gray, T. R.; Shakleya, D. M.; Huestis, M. A. A liquid chromatography tandem mass spectrometry method for the simultaneous quantification of 20 drugs of abuse and metabolites in human meconium. *Anal. Bioanal. Chem.*, 2009, 393, 1977–90.

[432] Concheiro, M.; Jones, H. E.; Johnson, R. E.; et al. Maternal buprenorphine dose, placenta buprenorphine and metabolite concentrations and neonatal outcomes. *Ther. Drug Monit.*, 2010, 32(2), 206-15.

[433] Deshmukh, S. V.; Nanovskaya, T. N.; Ahmed, M. S.. Aromatase is the major enzyme metabolizing buprenorphine in human placenta. *J. Pharmacol. Exp. Ther.*, 2003, 306(3), 1099-105.

[434] Fokina, V. M.; Patrikeeva, S. L.; Zharikova, O. L.; et al. Transplacental transfer and metabolism of buprenorphine in preterm human placenta. *Am. J. Perinatol.*, 2011, 28(1), 25-32.

[435] Nekhayeva, I. A.; Nanovskaya, T. N.; Hankins, G. D.; et al. Role of human placental efflux transporter P-glycoprotein in the transfer of buprenorphine, levo-alpha-acetylmethadol, and paclitaxel. *Am. J. Perinatol.*, 2006, 23(7), 423-30.

[436] Concheiro-Guisan, M.; Shakleya, D. M.; Huestis, M. A. Simultaneous quantification of buprenorphine, norbuprenorphine, buprenorphine glucuronide, and norbuprenorphine glucuronide in human placenta by liquid chromatography mass spectrometry. *Anal. Bioanal. Chem.*, 2009, 394(2), 513-22.

[437] Gordon, A. L.; Lopatko, O. V.; Somogyi, A. A.; et al. (R)- and (S)-methadone and buprenorphine concentration ratios in maternal and umbilical cord plasma following chronic maintenance dosing in pregnancy. *Br. J. Clin. Pharmacol.*, 2010, 70(6), 895-902.

[438] Concheiro, M.; Jones, H.; Johnson, R. E.; et al. Confirmatory analysis of buprenorphine, norbuprenorphine, and glucuronide metabolites in plasma by LCMSMS. Application to umbilical cord plasma from buprenorphine-maintained pregnant women. *J. Chromatogr. B. Analyt. Technol. Biomed. Life Sci.*, 2010, 878(1), 13-20.

[439] Concheiro, M.; Jones, H. E.; Johnson, R. E.; et al. Umbilical cord monitoring of in utero drug exposure to buprenorphine and correlation with maternal dose and neonatal outcomes. *J. Anal. Toxicol.*, 2010, 34(8), 498-505.

In: Buprenorphine
Editor: Rosalina Bennet

ISBN: 978-1-63321-136-0

Chapter 2

THE EMERGING ROLE OF BUPRENORPHINE AS AN ANALGESIC

Mellar P. Davis*

The Harry R Horvitz Center for Palliative Medicine, Division of Solid Tumor, Taussig Cancer Institute, Cleveland Clinic, Cleveland, Ohio

ABSTRACT

Potent opioids have different efficacy, particularly opioids such as buprenorphine may have advantages due to unique pharmacodynamics and pharmacokinetics. Prospective studies have demonstrated the benefits to buprenorphine in several clinical situations. However, randomized control trials are few and far between and need to be done to demonstrate these advantages. Buprenorphine appears to be a safe potent opioid with few drug interactions and reduced risk for respiratory, cardiac, gastrointestinal, sexual and cognitive adverse effects. Certain populations and clinical situations favor the use of buprenorphine as a first line opioid.

Keywords: Buprenorphine, analgesia, pharmacodynamics, pharmacokinetics, respiratory depression, cognitive function, constipation, immunosuppression

---

* Corresponding author: Mellar P. Davis, Prof. of Medicine, Division of Solid Tumor Oncology, Taussig Cancer Institute, Cleveland Clinic, 9500 Euclid Ave., Cleveland Ohio, 44195, E-mail: DAVISM6@ccf.org, Telephone: 216-445-4622

INTRODUCTION

Recommendations for opioid analgesics when pain is severe include hydromorphone, fentanyl, methadone, morphine, oxycodone and buprenorphine [1]. Analgesic responses, G protein activation, intrinsic efficacy and downstream signaling appear to be different between opioids even though few have actually been compared by randomized clinical trials [2-6]. In addition few have been compared within clinical context and between patient characteristics (organ function, polypharmacy, type of pain, age, gender). How does one choose a first or second line opioid?

Certain factors favor one potent opioids over another. Previous responses or lack of response to a certain opioid (or adverse or lack of adverse effects) logically guide the clinician's choice. A personal history of substance abuse, type of pain, organ reserve, age, perhaps gender and clinical context play a major role in the choice of opioid. Finally side effect, profile, function and personal goals will also be important to certain individuals when choosing an opioid.

Drug interactions are increasingly important particularly among the elderly. Certain opioids have potentially dangerous interactions with other medications. For instance methadone impairs cardiac repolarization and drugs which delay methadone clearance may cause sudden death. In certain clinical situations, as an example, individuals in pain with a prolonged QTc interval on multiple medications, methadone may not be the best choice [7-13]. For individuals who are already immunosuppressed, morphine and fentanyl may worsen remaining immunocompetence [14-19]. Certain clinical situations favor certain opioids. Opioids may be given by multiple routes (also called versatility). Morphine can be given by mouth, per rectum, IV, subcutaneous, epidural and intrathecal, whereas oxycodone is limited at least in the United States to oral administration (though it can also be given per rectum). Individuals on morphine who developed nausea or dysphagia can be switched to parenteral morphine without loss of analgesia which may not be possible with oxycodone.

So what are the advantages to buprenorphine relative to other opioids? Buprenorphine is an old, yet new opioid. The parenteral form has been available for greater than 30 years in the United States, yet new in the form of transdermal patches, sublingual tablets and film. Sublingual buprenorphine has been combined with naloxone to reduce abuse [20]. Buprenorphine may be seen as one of a number of opioid choices to manage pain.

PHARMACODYNAMICS

This oriparvine morphine derivative has a cyclopropylmethyl group which results in a unique receptor binding spectrum. Buprenorphine is not only a mu and delta opioid receptor agonist but a kappa opioid receptor antagonist and an orphanin/nociceptin (ORL-1) receptor agonist [20-22]. In animal models and clinically buprenorphine is a full analgesic agonist without an analgesic ceiling effect [23]. The receptor binding spectrum provides some unique clinical benefits.

It is important to understand the complexity of opioid pharmacodynamics which explains unique responses despite activating the same mu receptor. Our understanding has changed over the last 10 years. Receptors are in a dynamic state of conformational flux. Opioid agonists stabilize the receptor in multiple unique active conformations which result in unique downstream signaling and receptor trafficking [6]. Downstream signaling includes G-protein, beta arrestin-2, and kinase activation and activation of gene transcription. Receptor density, cellular health, receptor phosphorylation, type of co-binding proteins bias downstream signaling initiated by opioid-receptor conformation stabilization [6]. Buprenorphine in particular activates a distinct set of G proteins, different from other potent opioids [24, 25]. Buprenorphine activates pertussis toxin resistant G proteins in contradistinction to morphine, methadone and fentanyl. Buprenorphine downstream signaling differs from methadone as measured by the timing of adenylyl cyclase activation [26]. Buprenorphine is uniquely a "chaperone" ligand which increases mu receptor expression [27].

Unlike morphine and fentanyl, buprenorphine analgesia is not reversed by intracerebroventricular naloxone. This means that analgesia is not completely dependent on mu receptors. ORL-1 activation blocks analgesic tolerance. This may be due to dampening rostral ventromedial medulla "on cell" activity which is responsible in part for pain facilitation [28-31]. Finally buprenorphine is a kappa receptor antagonist. Potent opioids cause the release of spinal dynorphin, an endogenous kappa agonist, which also cause central sensitization [32]. Hence, buprenorphine potentially reverses central sensitization and hyperalgesia caused by other potent opioids. Buprenorphine has local anesthetic activity. Buprenorphine blocks voltage-gated sodium channels with greater potency than lidocaine and bupivacaine and blocks generation of C fiber action potentials with greater potential than lidocaine [33].

Most potent opioids have a limited ability to block central sensitization. Uniquely, buprenorphine has pronounced anti-hyperalgesia compared with fentanyl [34]. As a result, buprenorphine may be as effective if not better at reducing neuropathic pain which is also frequently associated with central sensitization. Buprenorphine attenuates more pain types (bone pain, heat pain, and nerve-growth factor-induced soreness) than fentanyl in human experimental pain [35].

Pharmacokinetics

Buprenorphine is readily absorbed transdermal and sublingual. This is largely due to its lipophilicity (octanol: water partition coefficient of 2000). Sublingual bioavailability is 30-50% compared with parenteral buprenorphine. Sublingual buprenorphine blood levels peak at 2 hours, rapidly decline over 6 hours and then slowly decline over the next 16 hours [36]. The terminal half-life is prolonged by enterohepatic recirculation. In fact the half-life of sublingual buprenorphine exceeds that of IV buprenorphine for that reason and for the fact that sublingual buprenorphine is sequestered in sublingual glands and buccal fat pad. Buprenorphine is metabolized to a weak active metabolite, norbuprenorphine, by CYP 3A4 and CYP 2C8 and is further conjugated to norbuprenorphine-3-glucuronide. Buprenorphine is also directly conjugated to buprenorphine-3-glucuronide [37].

Buprenorphine-3-glucuronide has high affinity for mu, delta and ORL.-1 receptors but not kappa while norbuprenorphine-3-glucuronide has affinity for kappa and ORL-1 receptors but not mu or delta receptors. Neither buprenorphine nor its glucuronide influence the respiratory rate. Norbuprenorphine and norbuprenorphine-3-glucuronide can reduce tidal volume. Of the metabolites, only buprenorphine-3-glucuronide has small but clinically detectable analgesia [38]. In animal models, norbuprenorphine causes less antinociception than buprenorphine but is responsible for respiratory depression [39, 40]. Norbuprenorphine but not buprenorphine is a substrate for P-glycoprotein. This limits norbuprenorphine CNS penetration [41]. The parent drug and metabolites are largely excreted in bile and stool, drug clearance therefore is not dependent on renal function [42].

Buprenorphine and metabolites do not inhibit cytochromes at therapeutic doses and despite metabolism through various cytochromes (similar to methadone and fentanyl); buprenorphine has fewer drug interactions than methadone or fentanyl [43, 44].

BENEFITS TO BUPRENORPHINE

Analgesia

Buprenorphine is an effective analgesic, as effective as fentanyl, morphine and oxycodone. The need for opioid rotation is less with buprenorphine compared with morphine; the need to increased doses over time (the opioid escalation index) is less with buprenorphine than with fentanyl [45, 46]. Multiple randomized trials have demonstrated buprenorphine benefits in managing cancer and non-cancer pain [22]. Discontinuation for side effects is less than 10%. Consistent analgesia over 3-5 years is well documented [47, 48]. Buprenorphine is safe to use in pediatric patients; the majority experience pain relief [49]. Buprenorphine can used with other opioids in the perioperative setting without loss of analgesia [50]. Combinations of buprenorphine and fentanyl have additive analgesia [51]. Buprenorphine is effective in reducing neuropathic pain [52]. Neuropathic injury results in loss of pertussis toxin sensitive G proteins which are critical to morphine analgesia. Buprenorphine analgesia is not dependent on pertussis toxin sensitive G proteins [53, 54]. Theoretical benefits of buprenorphine for neuropathic pain need be confirmed in randomized trials comparing buprenorphine with other potent opioids.

SAFETY

Respiratory Depression

One of the greatest fears physicians have when prescribing opioids is respiratory depression. Buprenorphine is a partial agonist with a ceiling effect on respiratory depression but a full analgesic agonist [55-57]. In human experimental pain, a plateau in respiratory depression is observed when buprenorphine doses were increased from 0.2 mg per kilogram to 0.4 mg per kilogram but no ceiling to analgesia [56]. This mirrors events in animal models [57]. At the same time, when respiratory depression does occur, high bolus doses of naloxone (2 mg) and a continuous infusion of high doses (2-4 mg per hour) are needed to reverse respiratory depression [58]. This is due to buprenorphine and in particular norbuprenorphine half-life and secondarily to mu receptor affinity. However, respiratory depression is unusual with buprenorphine alone, but will occur with greater risk when combined with a benzodiazepine [59]. In animal models, the safety index of buprenorphine is 10 fold greater than fentanyl [60]. Safety in high risk populations such as those with COPD and central sleep apnea needs to be established in prospective trials.

Cognition

Individuals on methadone and buprenorphine maintenance have increased frequency of motor vehicle accident compared with the normal population. This may reflect an impulsive personality and not the opioid [61]. Individuals on buprenorphine (which are most often high doses) compared with healthy controls have similar psychomotor and cognitive performance, attention span, reaction times, vigilance and motor coordination [62, 63]. Buprenorphine has lower psychomotor adverse effects. [64-67]. Theoretically, this may be due to buprenorphine activation of limbic and mesolimbic circuitry, selective reduction in affective sensory discrimination and reduced putamen-sensory structure connectivity (as measured by blood oxygen level-dependent functional MRI) [68]. Though several groups have recommended the use of buprenorphine in the elderly in part due to its limited cognitive adverse effects, randomized trials will be necessary to validate this recommendation [68-70].

Gastrointestinal Toxicity

Constipation is a major opioid side effect Constipation is also caused by multiple non-opioid medications, inactivity, reduced fluid and food intake and cancer related complications. Opioids account for 25-50% of constipation in advanced cancer [71]. Constipation leads to other symptoms such as colic, abdominal pain, nausea, vomiting and anorexia. Only 1-5% of individuals on buprenorphine experience significant constipation [47]. Transdermal buprenorphine is significantly less constipating than morphine [72]. Unlike other opioids, buprenorphine does not cause spasm of the sphincter of Oddi [73]. However, buprenorphine increase is intracholedochal passage pressures transiently similar to other opioids [74, 75]. Buprenorphine does not appear to cause liver toxicity as demonstrated by elevations of transaminases [76]. Hence buprenorphine may be a reasonable opioid to use for those with pain and constipation or for those with biliary tract cancers or biliary or bowel obstruction. This needs to be validated with additional studies.

Cardiac Toxicity

Methadone is associated with a prolonged QTc interval, Torsades de pointes and sudden cardiac death. Risks are dose related [77]. Unlike methadone individuals on maintenance buprenorphine have QTC intervals almost always less than 450 ms [78, 79]. If the QTC interval is prolonged on buprenorphine, it is more likely due to hypokalemia than buprenorphine [80]. Switching from methadone to buprenorphine will normalize the QTc interval in those with a prolonged QTc interval on methadone [81-83]. It is for this reason that overdose mortality is lower with buprenorphine than methadone. This probably reflects reduced cardiac arrhythmia and a ceiling effect on respiratory depression [84]. Cancer patients are usually on multiple medications which potentially increase the risk of adverse drug interactions and cardiac toxicity. Cardiac comorbidities are common in this population since most cancer patients are elderly. Buprenorphine is potentially a safer drug to use than methadone due to reduced drug interactions, respiratory depression and cardiac toxicity.

Buprenorphine can cause hypotension in a subset of patients. In randomized trials of postoperative pain, compared with parenteral morphine, parenteral buprenorphine produced equivalent reductions in systolic and diastolic blood pressure [85, 86]. In a recent randomized trial comparing sublingual buprenorphine 0.4 mg with intravenous morphine 5 mg for patients with acute fractures, 4% of patients treated with buprenorphine developed hypotension compared with 18% of morphine treated patients. Hypotension on buprenorphine was seen within 30 minutes of administration and resolved by 60 minutes [97].

Immunosuppression

Morphine and fentanyl decrease interleukin-2 and interferon gamma, inhibit adaptive immunity, down-regulate natural killer cell function and cellular-humoral responses to infection [88]. Buprenorphine, unlike morphine and fentanyl, is not immunosuppressive [14]. Pain activates the hypothalamic-pituitary-adrenal (HPA) axis increasing cortisol levels and sympathetic tone resulting in further immunosuppression. In animal models, buprenorphine reduces post-surgical pain behaviors and experimental metastatic colonization compared with morphine and fentanyl [17]. Buprenorphine as maintenance therapy for addiction reverses the immunocompromise of heroin abuse.

Reduced Sexual Function and Hypogonadism

Chronic opioids are associated with hypogonadotropic hypogonadism, loss of libido, fatigue and over time osteoporosis, gynecomastia, infertility and reduced muscle mass and strength [88-90]. Men on maintenance buprenorphine have higher testosterone levels than those on methadone [92]. Transdermal buprenorphine reduces pain without producing hypogonadism or altering menstrual cycles in females [4]. As a result, buprenorphine potentially over time will have fewer adverse sexual and musculoskeletal side effects than other potent opioids. Randomized control trials will be needed to confirm these benefits.

Addiction

Opioids should be avoided or special precautions and co-management with an addiction specialist considered when treating pain in someone with a history of drug abuse or addiction. Buprenorphine can produce rewarding effects similar to other potent opioids when tested in morphine and buprenorphine maintained addicts [95-98]. Buprenorphine, in approximately 20-27% of individuals on maintenance therapy, is diverted or abused; there has been an increase in abuse from 2005 to 2009 [99-103]. Buprenorphine-naloxone, however, blocks the rewarding effects of other opioids such as oxycodone and heroin in a dose-dependent fashion [104-106]. A significant reason for the diversion of buprenorphine is to prevent withdrawal when heroin or other street drugs are not available and as self-treatment for addiction [107-109]. Buprenorphine is the primary IV drug abused in only 10% of addicted individuals and is the least abused opioid in the United States [108, 110-114]. Abuse is no greater than that observed for the unscheduled drug tramadol and much less than the Schedule II drugs methadone and oxycodone [116]. The euphoric effects in non-addicted individuals are lower with buprenorphine than other potent opioids [108, 113, 116]. Opioid-related deaths are lower with buprenorphine than with methadone. IV buprenorphine abusers are less likely to share needles, are likely to take fewer injections and are or more likely attempting self-treatment or avoiding withdrawal. They are less likely to develop HIV infections [108, 118-120]. The abuse prevalence of buprenorphine therefore is not simply related to the biological properties of the drug but to a variety of social, culture and economic forces [105].

For Whom Should One Consider Buprenorphine As a First or Second Line Opioid?

Various populations and clinical scenarios are considered appropriate for buprenorphine. Individuals with chronic pain, cancer pain and a family history or personal history of drug abuse or addiction opioids should be avoided, buprenorphine may be considered as a first line opioid for reasons discussed above. Buprenorphine is available in combination with naloxone which prevents illicit route conversion. There is greater safety with buprenorphine than with methadone. There is also evidence that buprenorphine, when used to manage withdrawal symptoms does not produce either respiratory depression or a psychological "high" [121].

Individuals with dysphagia or bowel obstruction are candidates for sublingual buprenorphine or transdermal fentanyl or buprenorphine as a first line opioid. Sublingual buprenorphine is one of the two (methadone) long-acting sublingual opioids and allows clinicians to manage pain with few doses per day without the need for parenteral infusions or computer activated delivery devices (CADD pumps). In countries where transdermal buprenorphine is available, conversion from parenteral to transdermal buprenorphine is an alternative approach.

Individuals with unstable renal function, progressive renal failure or who are on dialyses are at risk for opioid toxicity with most potent opioids and should receive buprenorphine as first-line analgesia for severe to moderate pain. Buprenorphine is the safest of the opioids to use in renal failure. In addition buprenorphine is ideal to use in the intensive care setting, for those with multiple organ failure [122, 123].

Opioids in the elderly are associated with a significant risk of cognitive toxicity and falls and the elderly should be considered for front-line buprenorphine [69]. Buprenorphine pharmacokinetics are not different in the elderly compared with younger patients [124]. Buprenorphine benefits for those over the age of 65 years are equivalent to younger individuals [70].

Buprenorphine is the only opioid not associated with an increased falls risk in the elderly [125].

Buprenorphine preserves testosterone and estrogen levels and better maintains libido than other opioids [95-98]. This is distinctly different than other potent opioids [89, 126-129]. Buprenorphine should be considered as a front-line opioid in men who wished to maintain sexual function while receiving opioid analgesics.

Buprenorphine is a reasonable first choice for those individuals with heart disease and a prolonged QTc interval. Many of these individuals are on multiple medications which increase the risk of adverse drug-drug interactions and QTc prolongation. Buprenorphine has a reduced risk of adverse opioid drug interactions and will be just as effective as other opioids in reducing pain [130].

Buprenorphine should be considered as a first or second line opioid when managing neuropathic pain [131-137]. The unique anti-hyperalgesia properties of buprenorphine lend itself to managing neuropathic pain unresponsive to other potent opioids [34].

Buprenorphine should be used with caution in those with severe liver disease. Buprenorphine glucuronides can accumulate and is an active metabolite. In normal individuals buprenorphine glucuronide contributes only a small amount to analgesia but with accumulation may become clinically important. Norbuprenorphine-3-glucuronide contributes to respiratory depression [38].

Buprenorphine appears to be safe when administered with drugs that inhibit CYP3A4; there is little pharmacokinetic interactions between buprenorphine and HIV medications unlike oxycodone, fentanyl and methadone [44, 138]. Since most HIV infection in Eastern Europe and Asia is related to IV drug abuse, buprenorphine would be an excellent first line choice to manage pain in this population [108].

The Clinical Use of Buprenorphine

For acute pain, parenteral (IV or subcutaneous) buprenorphine can be used. The equianalgesic dose ratio of buprenorphine to fentanyl is 0.8-0.6 (fentanyl 25 mcg per hour is equivalent to buprenorphine 35 mcg per hour). Buprenorphine 35 mcg per hour is approximately equivalent to parenteral morphine 1 mg an hour. The oral morphine to buprenorphine ratio is 70-1. Starting doses for the opioid naïve should be 20-25 mcg per hour. Because of the long half-life, doses should not be changed more frequently than every 48 hours. Conversion from parenteral buprenorphine to sublingual should be done using a 1-2 ratio and from parenteral (subcutaneous or IV) to transdermal is 1-1.The variability of buprenorphine absorption from the transdermal patch means that doses may need to be adjusted after converting to the patch. The same is true when converting from parenteral to sublingual buprenorphine. A new sublingual buprenorphine-naloxone film is available as an alternative to tablets. The sublingual film is dose equivalent to the tablets and has comparable clinical outcomes [140]. Transdermal buprenorphine patches in the United States are approved for moderate pain only and are available in 5, 10 and 20 mcg patches which are changed weekly [140]. Application site reactions occur in 24%, most (98%) of reactions are mild to moderate with only 4% discontinuing buprenorphine due to applications site toxicity. The applications site needs to be rotated [141].

CONCLUSION

Buprenorphine is a unique opioid with several advantages over commonly used potent opioids depending upon the clinical situation. It is important that clinicians become knowledgeable about buprenorphine in order to improve their pain management skills.

Future Perspective

Buprenorphine is now a very popular drug for maintenance therapy [47, 148]. There has been a significant amount of work done in the past which has demonstrated buprenorphine benefits in managing multiple different pains including cancer related pain and neuropathic pain [142, 143].

The World Health Organization that has added buprenorphine to the list of complimentary medication in the 14th edition of the Model List of Essential Medicines [144]. The rise in opioid deaths (particularly methadone), the rise in opioid abuse and the safety factor of buprenorphine makes it quite an attractive opioid to use both in the cancer population, HIV patients and in those unfortunate individuals with non-cancer related pain who may benefit from opioid analgesics. Buprenorphine equianalgesia has been established with methadone and fentanyl such that rotation to buprenorphine is easily accomplished [22, 145-148]. Buprenorphine use therefore is likely to increase over the next 5-10 years and the use of methadone decrease as clinicians become comfortable with the use of buprenorphine.

Key Points

- Buprenorphine activates a distinct set of G proteins, downstream signaling differs from methadone, uniquely acts a "chaperone" ligand which increases mu receptor expression, activates ORL-1, blocks analgesic tolerance, and is a kappa receptor antagonist.
- Buprenorphine is readily absorbed transdermal and sublingual. Sublingual bioavailability is 30-50%. Buprenorphine is metabolized to a weak active metabolite, norbuprenorphine, by CYP 3A4 and CYP 2C8 and conjugated to norbuprenorphine-3-glucuronide
- Buprenorphine is an effective analgesic, as effective as fentanyl, morphine and oxycodone. The need for opioid rotation is less with buprenorphine compared with morphine; the need to increased doses over time (the opioid escalation index) is less with buprenorphine than with fentanyl.
- Respiratory depression is unusual with buprenorphine alone, but will occur with greater risk when combined with a benzodiazepine
- Switching from methadone to buprenorphine will normalize the QTc interval in those with a prolonged QTc interval on methadone
- Buprenorphine can cause hypotension in a subset of patients similar to that of opioids
- Abuse is no greater than that observed for the unscheduled drug tramadol and much less than the Schedule II drugs methadone and oxycodone. The euphoric effects in non-addicted individuals are lower with buprenorphine than other potent opioids. Abuse and diversion may be related to prevention of withdrawal symptoms and for self-treatment of addiction
- Buprenorphine should be considered a first line drugs for those in overt renal failure, family or personal history of drug abuse or addiction, for preservation of sexual function, for cancer or neuropathic pain, for the elderly, for those who require a long-acting sublingual opioid to avoid parenteral injections, for the immunosuppressed and for those on highly active antiretroviral medications.

- Buprenorphine should be used with caution in those with significant liver disease.

References

[1] Caraceni A, Hanks G, Kaasa S et al.: Use of opioid analgesics in the treatment of cancer pain: evidence-based recommendations from the EAPC. *Lancet Oncol.* 13(2), e58-68 (2012).

[2] Garzon J, Garcia-Espana A, Sanchez-Blazquez P: Opioids binding mu and delta receptors exhibit diverse efficacy in the activation of Gi2 and G(x/z) transducer proteins in mouse periaqueductal gray matter. *The Journal of pharmacology and experimental therapeutics* 281(1), 549-557 (1997).

[3] Garzon J, Martinez-Pena Y, Sanchez-Blazquez P: Dissimilar efficacy of opioids to produce mu-mediated analgesia: role of Gx/z and Gi2 transducer proteins. *Life sciences* 55(11), PL205-212 (1994).

[4] Sanchez-Blazquez P, Garzon J: Pertussis toxin differentially reduces the efficacy of opioids to produce supraspinal analgesia in the mouse. *European journal of pharmacology* 152(3), 357-361 (1988).

[5] Kelly E: Efficacy and ligand bias at the mu-opioid receptor. *British journal of pharmacology* 169(7), 1430-1446 (2013).

[6] Kenakin T: New concepts in pharmacological efficacy at 7TM receptors: IUPHAR review 2. *British journal of pharmacology* 168(3), 554-575 (2013).

[7] Pani PP, Trogu E, Maremmani I, Pacini M: QTc interval screening for cardiac risk in methadone treatment of opioid dependence. *Cochrane database of systematic reviews* 6, CD008939 (2013).

[8] Winton JC, Twilla JD: Sudden cardiac arrest in a patient on chronic methadone after the addition of azithromycin. *The American journal of the medical sciences* 345(2), 160-162 (2013).

[9] Lin C, Somberg T, Molnar J, Somberg J: The effects of chiral isolates of methadone on the cardiac potassium channel IKr. *Cardiology* 113(1), 59-65 (2009).

[10] Slotkin TA, Weigel SJ, Seidler FJ, Whitmore WL: Toxic effects of maternal methadone administration on cardiac development in the neonatal rat: potential participation of altered polyamine levels in growth impairment. *Toxicology letters* 14(3-4), 131-135 (1982).

[11] Fareed A, Patil D, Scheinberg K *et al.*: Comparison of QTc Interval Prolongation for Patients in Methadone Versus Buprenorphine Maintenance Treatment: A 5-Year Follow-Up. *Journal of addictive diseases* 32(3), 244-251 (2013).

[12] Abramson DW, Quinn DK, Stern TA: Methadone-Associated QTc Prolongation: A Case Report and Review of the Literature. *Primary care companion to the Journal of clinical psychiatry* 10(6), 470-476 (2008).

[13] Kornick CA, Kilborn MJ, Santiago-Palma J et al.: QTc interval prolongation associated with intravenous methadone. *Pain* 105(3), 499-506 (2003).

[14] Sacerdote P: Opioid-induced immunosuppression. *Current opinion in supportive and palliative care* 2(1), 14-18 (2008).

[15] Sacerdote P, Franchi S, Gerra G, Leccese V, Panerai AE, Somaini L: Buprenorphine and methadone maintenance treatment of heroin addicts preserves immune function. *Brain, behavior, and immunity* 22(4), 606-613 (2008).

[16] Shavit Y, Ben-Eliyahu S, Zeidel A, Beilin B: Effects of fentanyl on natural killer cell activity and on resistance to tumor metastasis in rats. Dose and timing study. *Neuroimmunomodulation* 11(4), 255-260 (2004).

[17] Franchi S, Panerai AE, Sacerdote P: Buprenorphine ameliorates the effect of surgery on hypothalamus-pituitary-adrenal axis, natural killer cell activity and metastatic colonization in rats in comparison with morphine or fentanyl treatment. *Brain, behavior, and immunity* 21(6), 767-774 (2007).

[18] Martucci C, Panerai AE, Sacerdote P: Chronic fentanyl or buprenorphine infusion in the mouse: similar analgesic profile but different effects on immune responses. *Pain* 110(1-2), 385-392 (2004).

[19] Gomez-Flores R, Weber RJ: Differential effects of buprenorphine and morphine on immune and neuroendocrine functions following acute administration in the rat mesencephalon periaqueductal gray. *Immunopharmacology* 48(2), 145-156 (2000).

[20] Davis MP: Twelve reasons for considering buprenorphine as a frontline analgesic in the management of pain. *The journal of supportive oncology* 10(6), 209-219 (2012).

[21] Bloms-Funke P, Gillen C, Schuettler AJ, Wnendt S: Agonistic effects of the opioid buprenorphine on the nociceptin/OFQ receptor. *Peptides* 21(7), 1141-1146 (2000).

[22] Pergolizzi J, Aloisi AM, Dahan A et al.: Current knowledge of buprenorphine and its unique pharmacological profile. *Pain practice : the official journal of World Institute of Pain* 10(5), 428-450 (2010).
[23] Christoph T, Kogel B, Schiene K, Meen M, De Vry J, Friderichs E: Broad analgesic profile of buprenorphine in rodent models of acute and chronic pain. *Eur. J. Pharmacol.* 507(1-3), 87-98 (2005).
[24] Ocana M, Del Pozo E, Barrios M, Baeyens JM: Subgroups among mu-opioid receptor agonists distinguished by ATP-sensitive K+ channel-acting drugs. *Br. J. Pharmacol.* 114(6), 1296-1302 (1995).
[25] Saidak Z, Blake-Palmer K, Hay DL, Northup JK, Glass M: Differential activation of G-proteins by mu-opioid receptor agonists. *Br. J. Pharmacol.* 147(6), 671-680 (2006).
[26] Lee CW, Yan JY, Chiang YC et al.: Differential pharmacological actions of methadone and buprenorphine in human embryonic kidney 293 cells coexpressing human mu-opioid and opioid receptor-like 1 receptors. *Neurochemical research* 36(11), 2008-2021 (2011).
[27] Zaki PA, Keith DE, Jr., Brine GA, Carroll FI, Evans CJ: Ligand-induced changes in surface mu-opioid receptor number: relationship to G protein activation? *J. Pharmacol. Exp. Ther.* 292(3), 1127-1134 (2000).
[28] Cowan A, Doxey JC, Harry EJ: The animal pharmacology of buprenorphine, an oripavine analgesic agent. *Br. J. Pharmacol.* 60(4), 547-554 (1977).
[29] Cowan A, Lewis JW, Macfarlane IR: Agonist and antagonist properties of buprenorphine, a new antinociceptive agent. *Br. J. Pharmacol.* 60(4), 537-545 (1977).
[30] Heinricher MM: Orphanin FQ/nociceptin: from neural circuitry to behavior. *Life Sci.* 73(6), 813-822 (2003).
[31] Heinricher MM, Mcgaraughty S, Grandy DK: Circuitry underlying antiopioid actions of orphanin FQ in the rostral ventromedial medulla. *J. Neurophysiol* 78(6), 3351-3358 (1997).
[32] Vanderah TW, Gardell LR, Burgess SE et al.: Dynorphin promotes abnormal pain and spinal opioid antinociceptive tolerance. *J. Neurosci.* 20(18), 7074-7079 (2000).
[33] Leffler A, Frank G, Kistner K et al.: Local anesthetic-like inhibition of voltage-gated Na(+) channels by the partial mu-opioid receptor agonist buprenorphine. *Anesthesiology* 116(6), 1335-1346 (2012).
[34] Koppert W, Ihmsen H, Korber N et al.: Different profiles of buprenorphine-induced analgesia and antihyperalgesia in a human pain model. *Pain* 118(1-2), 15-22 (2005).

[35] Andresen T, Upton RN, Foster DJ, Christrup LL, Arendt-Nielsen L, Drewes AM: Pharmacokinetic/pharmacodynamic relationships of transdermal buprenorphine and fentanyl in experimental human pain models. *Basic & clinical pharmacology & toxicology* 108(4), 274-284 (2011).

[36] Kuhlman JJ, Jr., Lalani S, Magluilo J, Jr., Levine B, Darwin WD: Human pharmacokinetics of intravenous, sublingual, and buccal buprenorphine. *J Anal Toxicol* 20(6), 369-378 (1996).

[37] Picard N, Cresteil T, Djebli N, Marquet P: In vitro metabolism study of buprenorphine: evidence for new metabolic pathways. *Drug Metab Dispos* 33(5), 689-695 (2005).

[38] Brown SM, Holtzman M, Kim T, Kharasch ED: Buprenorphine metabolites, buprenorphine-3-glucuronide and norbuprenorphine-3-glucuronide, are biologically active. *Anesthesiology* 115(6), 1251-1260 (2011).

[39] Huang P, Kehner GB, Cowan A, Liu-Chen LY: Comparison of pharmacological activities of buprenorphine and norbuprenorphine: norbuprenorphine is a potent opioid agonist. *J. Pharmacol. Exp. Ther.* 297(2), 688-695 (2001).

[40] Ohtani M, Kotaki H, Nishitateno K, Sawada Y, Iga T: Kinetics of respiratory depression in rats induced by buprenorphine and its metabolite, norbuprenorphine. *J. Pharmacol. Exp. Ther.* 281(1), 428-433 (1997).

[41] Brown SM, Campbell SD, Crafford A, Regina KJ, Holtzman MJ, Kharasch ED: P-glycoprotein is a major determinant of norbuprenorphine brain exposure and antinociception. *J. Pharmacol. Exp. Ther.* 343(1), 53-61 (2012).

[42] Ohtani M, Kotaki H, Uchino K, Sawada Y, Iga T: Pharmacokinetic analysis of enterohepatic circulation of buprenorphine and its active metabolite, norbuprenorphine, in rats. *Drug Metab. Dispos.* 22(1), 2-7 (1994).

[43] Zhang W, Ramamoorthy Y, Tyndale RF, Sellers EM: Interaction of buprenorphine and its metabolite norbuprenorphine with cytochromes p450 in vitro. *Drug Metab. Dispos.* 31(6), 768-772 (2003).

[44] Kapil RP, Cipriano A, Michels GH *et al.*: Effect of ketoconazole on the pharmacokinetic profile of buprenorphine following administration of a once-weekly buprenorphine transdermal system. *Clinical drug investigation* 32(9), 583-592 (2012).

[45] Corli O, Montanari M, Deandrea S, Greco MT, Villani W, Apolone G: An exploratory analysis on the effectiveness of four strong opioids in patients with cancer pain. *Pain Med.* 13(7), 897-907 (2012).

[46] Mitra F, Chowdhury S, Shelley M, Williams G: A feasibility study of transdermal buprenorphine versus transdermal fentanyl in the long-term management of persistent non-cancer pain. *Pain medicine* 14(1), 75-83 (2013).

[47] Likar R, Kayser H, Sittl R: Long-term management of chronic pain with transdermal buprenorphine: a multicenter, open-label, follow-up study in patients from three short-term clinical trials. *Clinical therapeutics* 28(6), 943-952 (2006).

[48] Poulain P, Denier W, Douma J *et al.*: Efficacy and safety of transdermal buprenorphine: a randomized, placebo-controlled trial in 289 patients with severe cancer pain. *J. Pain Symptom Manage* 36(2), 117-125 (2008).

[49] Ruggiero A, Coccia P, Arena R *et al.*: Efficacy and safety of transdermal buprenorphine in the management of children with cancer-related pain. *Pediatr Blood Cancer* 60(3), 433-437 (2013).

[50] Macintyre P, Russell R, Usher K, Gaughwin M, Huxtable C: Pain relief and opioid requirements in the first 24 hours after surgery in patients taking buprenorphine and methadone opioid substitution therapy. *Anaesth Intensive Care* 41(2), 222-230 (2013).

[51] Troster A, Ihmsen H, Singler B, Filitz J, Koppert W: Interaction of fentanyl and buprenorphine in an experimental model of pain and central sensitization in human volunteers. *The Clinical journal of pain* 28(8), 705-711 (2012).

[52] Penza P, Campanella A, Martini A *et al.*: Short- and intermediate-term efficacy of buprenorphine TDS in chronic painful neuropathies. *J. Peripher. Nerv. Syst.* 13(4), 283-288 (2008).

[53] Mccormack K, Prather P, Chapleo C: Some new insights into the effects of opioids in phasic and tonic nociceptive tests. *Pain* 78(2), 79-98 (1998).

[54] Womer DE, Delapp NW, Shannon HE: Intrathecal pertussis toxin produces hyperalgesia and allodynia in mice. *Pain* 70(2-3), 223-228 (1997).

[55] Dahan A: Opioid-induced respiratory effects: new data on buprenorphine. *Palliat Med.* 20 Suppl 1, s3-8 (2006).

[56] Dahan A, Yassen A, Romberg R *et al.*: Buprenorphine induces ceiling in respiratory depression but not in analgesia. *Br. J. Anaesth.* 96(5), 627-632 (2006).

[57] Dahan A, Yassen A, Bijl H *et al.*: Comparison of the respiratory effects of intravenous buprenorphine and fentanyl in humans and rats. *British journal of anaesthesia* 94(6), 825-834 (2005).

[58] Sarton E, Teppema L, Dahan A: Naloxone reversal of opioid-induced respiratory depression with special emphasis on the partial agonist/antagonist buprenorphine. *Adv. Exp. Med. Biol.* 605, 486-491 (2008).

[59] Reynaud M, Tracqui A, Petit G, Potard D, Courty P: Six deaths linked to misuse of buprenorphine-benzodiazepine combinations. *Am. J. Psychiatry* 155(3), 448-449 (1998).

[60] Yassen A, Olofsen E, Kan J, Dahan A, Danhof M: Pharmacokinetic-pharmacodynamic modeling of the effectiveness and safety of buprenorphine and fentanyl in rats. *Pharmaceutical research* 25(1), 183-193 (2008).

[61] Strand MC, Fjeld B, Arnestad M, Morland J: Can patients receiving opioid maintenance therapy safely drive? A systematic review of epidemiological and experimental studies on driving ability with a focus on concomitant methadone or buprenorphine administration. *Traffic injury prevention* 14(1), 26-38 (2013).

[62] Dagtekin O, Gerbershagen HJ, Wagner W, Petzke F, Radbruch L, Sabatowski R: Assessing cognitive and psychomotor performance under long-term treatment with transdermal buprenorphine in chronic noncancer pain patients. *Anesthesia and analgesia* 105(5), 1442-1448, table of contents (2007).

[63] Shmygalev S, Damm M, Weckbecker K, Berghaus G, Petzke F, Sabatowski R: The impact of long-term maintenance treatment with buprenorphine on complex psychomotor and cognitive function. *Drug and alcohol dependence* 117(2-3), 190-197 (2011).

[64] Kress HG: Clinical update on the pharmacology, efficacy and safety of transdermal buprenorphine. *Eur. J. Pain* 13(3), 219-230 (2009).

[65] Singhal A, Tripathi BM, Pal HR, Jena R, Jain R: Effect of buprenorphine on psychomotor functions in patients on buprenorphine maintenance. *Journal of opioid management* 4(1), 41-47 (2008).

[66] Soyka M, Hock B, Kagerer S, Lehnert R, Limmer C, Kuefner H: Less impairment on one portion of a driving-relevant psychomotor battery in buprenorphine-maintained than in methadone-maintained patients:

results of a randomized clinical trial. *Journal of clinical psychopharmacology* 25(5), 490-493 (2005).

[67] Upadhyay J, Anderson J, Baumgartner R *et al.*: Modulation of CNS pain circuitry by intravenous and sublingual doses of buprenorphine. *Neuroimage* 59(4), 3762-3773 (2012).

[68] Van Ojik AL, Jansen PA, Brouwers JR, Van Roon EN: Treatment of chronic pain in older people: evidence-based choice of strong-acting opioids. *Drugs Aging* 29(8), 615-625 (2012).

[69] Pergolizzi J, Boger RH, Budd K *et al.*: Opioids and the management of chronic severe pain in the elderly: consensus statement of an International Expert Panel with focus on the six clinically most often used World Health Organization Step III opioids (buprenorphine, fentanyl, hydromorphone, methadone, morphine, oxycodone). *Pain practice : the official journal of World Institute of Pain* 8(4), 287-313 (2008).

[70] Muriel Villoria C, Perez-Castejon Garrote JM, Sanchez Magro I, Neira Alvarez M: [Effectiveness and safety of transdermal buprenorphine for chronic pain treatment in the elderly: a prospective observational study]. *Med Clin (Barc)* 128(6), 204-210 (2007).

[71] Sykes NP: The pathogenesis of constipation. *J. Support Oncol.* 4(5), 213-218 (2006).

[72] Tassinari D, Sartori S, Tamburini E *et al.*: Adverse effects of transdermal opiates treating moderate-severe cancer pain in comparison to long-acting morphine: a meta-analysis and systematic review of the literature. *J. Palliat Med.* 11(3), 492-501 (2008).

[73] Staritz M, Poralla T, Manns M, Meyer Zum Buschenfelde KH: Effect of modern analgesic drugs (tramadol, pentazocine, and buprenorphine) on the bile duct sphincter in man. *Gut.* 27(5), 567-569 (1986).

[74] Pausawasdi S, Kanjanapitak A, Kanjanapanjapol S: The effect of buprenorphine and morphine on intraluminal pressure of the common bile duct. *Journal of the Medical Association of Thailand = Chotmaihet thangphaet* 67(6), 329-333 (1984).

[75] Tigerstedt I, Turunen M, Tammisto T, Hastbacka J: The effect of buprenorphine and oxycodone on the intracholedochal passage pressure. *Acta anaesthesiologica Scandinavica* 25(2), 99-102 (1981).

[76] Saxon AJ, Ling W, Hillhouse M *et al.*: Buprenorphine/Naloxone and methadone effects on laboratory indices of liver health: a randomized trial. *Drug and alcohol dependence* 128(1-2), 71-76 (2013).

[77] Krantz MJ, Martin J, Stimmel B, Mehta D, Haigney MC: QTc interval screening in methadone treatment. *Annals of internal medicine* 150(6), 387-395 (2009).

[78] Anchersen K, Clausen T, Gossop M, Hansteen V, Waal H: Prevalence and clinical relevance of corrected QT interval prolongation during methadone and buprenorphine treatment: a mortality assessment study. *Addiction* 104(6), 993-999 (2009).

[79] Athanasos P, Farquharson AL, Compton P, Psaltis P, Hay J: Electrocardiogram characteristics of methadone and buprenorphine maintained subjects. *J. Addict Dis.* 27(3), 31-35 (2008).

[80] Stallvik M, Nordstrand B, Kristensen O, Bathen J, Skogvoll E, Spigset O: Corrected QT interval during treatment with methadone and buprenorphine--relation to doses and serum concentrations. *Drug Alcohol Depend* 129(1-2), 88-93 (2013).

[81] Krantz MJ, Lowery CM, Martell BA, Gourevitch MN, Arnsten JH: Effects of methadone on QT-interval dispersion. *Pharmacotherapy* 25(11), 1523-1529 (2005).

[82] Krantz MJ, Garcia JA, Mehler PS: Effects of buprenorphine on cardiac repolarization in a patient with methadone-related torsade de pointes. *Pharmacotherapy* 25(4), 611-614 (2005).

[83] Esses JL, Rosman J, Do LT, Schweitzer P, Hanon S: Successful transition to buprenorphine in a patient with methadone-induced torsades de pointes. *J. Interv. Card Electrophysiol.* 23(2), 117-119 (2008).

[84] Bell JR, Butler B, Lawrance A, Batey R, Salmelainen P: Comparing overdose mortality associated with methadone and buprenorphine treatment. *Drug Alcohol Depend* 104(1-2), 73-77 (2009).

[85] Tigerstedt I, Tammisto T: Double-blind, multiple-dose comparison of buprenorphine and morphine in postoperative pain. *Acta anaesthesiologica Scandinavica* 24(6), 462-468 (1980).

[86] Weiss P, Ritz R: [Analgesic effect and side-effects of buprenorphine in acute coronary heart disease. A randomized double-blind comparison with morphine]. *Anasthesie, Intensivtherapie, Notfallmedizin* 23(6), 309-312 (1988).

[87] Jalili M, Fathi M, Moradi-Lakeh M, Zehtabchi S: Sublingual buprenorphine in acute pain management: a double-blind randomized clinical trial. *Annals of emergency medicine* 59(4), 276-280 (2012).

[88] Sacerdote P: Opioids and the immune system. *Palliative medicine* 20 Suppl 1, s9-15 (2006).

[89] Paice JA, Penn RD, Ryan WG: Altered sexual function and decreased testosterone in patients receiving intraspinal opioids. *Journal of pain and symptom management* 9(2), 126-131 (1994).

[90] Aloisi AM, Buonocore M, Merlo L et al.: Chronic pain therapy and hypothalamic-pituitary-adrenal axis impairment. *Psychoneuro endocrinology* 36(7), 1032-1039 (2011).

[91] Bliesener N, Albrecht S, Schwager A, Weckbecker K, Lichtermann D, Klingmuller D: Plasma testosterone and sexual function in men receiving buprenorphine maintenance for opioid dependence. *The Journal of clinical endocrinology and metabolism* 90(1), 203-206 (2005).

[92] Hallinan R, Byrne A, Agho K, Mcmahon C, Tynan P, Attia J: Erectile dysfunction in men receiving methadone and buprenorphine maintenance treatment. *The journal of sexual medicine* 5(3), 684-692 (2008).

[93] Hallinan R, Byrne A, Agho K, Mcmahon CG, Tynan P, Attia J: Hypogonadism in men receiving methadone and buprenorphine maintenance treatment. *International journal of andrology* 32(2), 131-139 (2009).

[94] Aurilio C, Ceccarelli I, Pota V *et al.*: Endocrine and behavioural effects of transdermal buprenorphine in pain-suffering women of different reproductive ages. *Endocrine journal* 58(12), 1071-1078 (2011).

[95] Comer SD, Collins ED, Fischman MW: Intravenous buprenorphine self-administration by detoxified heroin abusers. *The Journal of pharmacology and experimental therapeutics* 301(1), 266-276 (2002).

[96] Comer SD, Collins ED: Self-administration of intravenous buprenorphine and the buprenorphine/naloxone combination by recently detoxified heroin abusers. *The Journal of pharmacology and experimental therapeutics* 303(2), 695-703 (2002).

[97] Comer SD, Sullivan MA, Walker EA: Comparison of intravenous buprenorphine and methadone self-administration by recently detoxified heroin-dependent individuals. *The Journal of pharmacology and experimental therapeutics* 315(3), 1320-1330 (2005).

[98] Comer SD, Sullivan MA, Whittington RA, Vosburg SK, Kowalczyk WJ: Abuse liability of prescription opioids compared to heroin in morphine-maintained heroin abusers. *Neuropsychopharmacology : official publication of the American College of Neuropsychopharmacology* 33(5), 1179-1191 (2008).

[99] Larance B, Degenhardt L, Lintzeris N *et al.*: Post-marketing surveillance of buprenorphine-naloxone in Australia: diversion, injection and adherence with supervised dosing. *Drug and alcohol dependence* 118(2-3), 265-273 (2011).

[100] Larance B, Ambekar A, Azim T *et al.*: The availability, diversion and injection of pharmaceutical opioids in South Asia. *Drug and alcohol review* 30(3), 246-254 (2011).

[101] Larance B, Degenhardt L, Lintzeris N, Winstock A, Mattick R: Definitions related to the use of pharmaceutical opioids: extramedical use, diversion, non-adherence and aberrant medication-related behaviours. *Drug and alcohol review* 30(3), 236-245 (2011).

[102] Larance B, Degenhardt L, O'brien S *et al.*: Prescribers' perceptions of the diversion and injection of medication by opioid substitution treatment patients. *Drug and alcohol review* 30(6), 613-620 (2011).

[103] Johanson CE, Arfken CL, Di Menza S, Schuster CR: Diversion and abuse of buprenorphine: findings from national surveys of treatment patients and physicians. *Drug and alcohol dependence* 120(1-3), 190-195 (2012).

[104] Jones JD, Sullivan MA, Manubay J, Vosburg SK, Comer SD: The subjective, reinforcing, and analgesic effects of oxycodone in patients with chronic, non-malignant pain who are maintained on sublingual buprenorphine/naloxone. *Neuropsychopharmacology: official publication of the American College of Neuropsychopharmacology* 36(2), 411-422 (2011).

[105] Comer SD, Sullivan MA, Vosburg SK *et al.*: Abuse liability of intravenous buprenorphine/naloxone and buprenorphine alone in buprenorphine-maintained intravenous heroin abusers. *Addiction* 105(4), 709-718 (2010).

[106] Comer SD, Collins ED, Fischman MW: Buprenorphine sublingual tablets: effects on IV heroin self-administration by humans. *Psychopharmacology* 154(1), 28-37 (2001).

[107] Alho H, Sinclair D, Vuori E, Holopainen A: Abuse liability of buprenorphine-naloxone tablets in untreated IV drug users. *Drug and alcohol dependence* 88(1), 75-78 (2007).

[108] Yokell MA, Zaller ND, Green TC, Rich JD: Buprenorphine and buprenorphine/naloxone diversion, misuse, and illicit use: an international review. *Current drug abuse reviews* 4(1), 28-41 (2011).

[109] Bazazi AR, Yokell M, Fu JJ, Rich JD, Zaller ND: Illicit use of buprenorphine/naloxone among injecting and noninjecting opioid users. *Journal of addiction medicine* 5(3), 175-180 (2011).
[110] Aitken CK, Higgs PG, Hellard ME: Buprenorphine injection in Melbourne, Australia--an update. *Drug and alcohol review* 27(2), 197-199 (2008).
[111] Cicero TJ, Inciardi JA, Munoz A: Trends in abuse of Oxycontin and other opioid analgesics in the United States: 2002-2004. *The journal of pain: official journal of the American Pain Society* 6(10), 662-672 (2005).
[112] Smith MY, Schneider MF, Wentz A, Hughes A, Haddox JD, Dart R: Quantifying morbidity associated with the abuse and misuse of opioid analgesics: a comparison of two approaches. *Clinical toxicology* 45(1), 23-30 (2007).
[113] Schneider MF, Bailey JE, Cicero TJ *et al.*: Integrating nine prescription opioid analgesics and/or four signal detection systems to summarize statewide prescription drug abuse in the United States in 2007. *Pharmacoepidemiology and drug safety* 18(9), 778-790 (2009).
[114] Smith MY, Bailey JE, Woody GE, Kleber HD: Abuse of buprenorphine in the United States: 2003-2005. *Journal of addictive diseases* 26(3), 107-111 (2007).
[115] Cicero TJ, Inciardi JA: Potential for abuse of buprenorphine in office-based treatment of opioid dependence. *The New England journal of medicine* 353(17), 1863-1865 (2005).
[116] Orman JS, Keating GM: Spotlight on buprenorphine/naloxone in the treatment of opioid dependence. *CNS drugs* 23(10), 899-902 (2009).
[117] Johnson RE, Strain EC, Amass L: Buprenorphine: how to use it right. *Drug and alcohol dependence* 70(2 Suppl), S59-77 (2003).
[118] Walsh SL, Eissenberg T: The clinical pharmacology of buprenorphine: extrapolating from the laboratory to the clinic. *Drug and alcohol dependence* 70(2 Suppl), S13-27 (2003).
[119] Robinson SE: Buprenorphine: an analgesic with an expanding role in the treatment of opioid addiction. *CNS drug reviews* 8(4), 377-390 (2002).
[120] Kintz P: Deaths involving buprenorphine: a compendium of French cases. *Forensic science international* 121(1-2), 65-69 (2001).
[121] Welsh CJ, Suman M, Cohen A, Broyles L, Bennett M, Weintraub E: The use of intravenous buprenorphine for the treatment of opioid withdrawal in medically ill hospitalized patients. *Am. J. Addict* 11(2), 135-140 (2002).

[122] Gawrisch E, Cheng EY: Buprenorphine sedation of intensive care patients and ileus reversal. *Critical care medicine* 18(9), 1034-1036 (1990).

[123] Downing JW, Goodwin NM, Hicks J: The respiratory depressive effects of intravenous buprenorphine in patients in an intensive care unit. *South African medical journal = Suid-Afrikaanse tydskrif vir geneeskunde* 55(25), 1023-1027 (1979).

[124] Al-Tawil N, Odar-Cederlof I, Berggren AC, Johnson HE, Persson J: Pharmacokinetics of transdermal buprenorphine patch in the elderly. *European journal of clinical pharmacology* 69(2), 143-149 (2013).

[125] Vestergaard P, Rejnmark L, Mosekilde L: Fracture risk associated with the use of morphine and opiates. *J. Intern. Med.* 260(1), 76-87 (2006).

[126] Opioids and hypogonadism. *Prescrire international* 21(126), 98-99 (2012).

[127] Schneider J: Hypogonadism in men treated with chronic opioids. *Archives of physical medicine and rehabilitation* 89(7), 1414; author reply 1414 (2008).

[128] Rajagopal A, Vassilopoulou-Sellin R, Palmer JL, Kaur G, Bruera E: Symptomatic hypogonadism in male survivors of cancer with chronic exposure to opioids. *Cancer* 100(4), 851-858 (2004).

[129] Daniell HW: Hypogonadism in men consuming sustained-action oral opioids. *The journal of pain : official journal of the American Pain Society* 3(5), 377-384 (2002).

[130] Mistry M, Houston JB: Glucuronidation in vitro and in vivo. Comparison of intestinal and hepatic conjugation of morphine, naloxone, and buprenorphine. *Drug Metab. Dispos.* 15(5), 710-717 (1987).

[131] Licina L, Hamsher C, Lautenschager K, Dhanjal S, Williams N, Spevak C: Buprenorphine/Naloxone therapy for opioid refractory neuropathic pain following traumatic amputation: a case series. *Military medicine* 178(7), e858-861 (2013).

[132] Weiner M, Sarantopoulos C, Gordon E: Transdermal buprenorphine controls central neuropathic pain. *Journal of opioid management* 8(6), 414-415 (2012).

[133] Guetti C, Angeletti C, Marinangeli F et al.: Transdermal buprenorphine for central neuropathic pain: clinical reports. *Pain practice : the official journal of World Institute of Pain* 11(5), 446-452 (2011).

[134] Induru RR, Davis MP: Buprenorphine for neuropathic pain--targeting hyperalgesia. *The American journal of hospice & palliative care* 26(6), 470-473 (2009).

[135] Hans G: Buprenorphine--a review of its role in neuropathic pain. *Journal of opioid management* 3(4), 195-206 (2007).

[136] Likar R, Sittl R: Transdermal buprenorphine for treating nociceptive and neuropathic pain: four case studies. *Anesthesia and analgesia* 100(3), 781-785, table of contents (2005).

[137] Kouya PF, Hao JX, Xu XJ: Buprenorphine alleviates neuropathic pain-like behaviors in rats after spinal cord and peripheral nerve injury. *European journal of pharmacology* 450(1), 49-53 (2002).

[138] Gruber VA, Rainey PM, Moody DE et al.: Interactions between buprenorphine and the protease inhibitors darunavir-ritonavir and fosamprenavir-ritonavir. *Clinical infectious diseases : an official publication of the Infectious Diseases Society of America* 54(3), 414-423 (2012).

[139] Lintzeris N, Leung SY, Dunlop AJ *et al.*: A randomised controlled trial of sublingual buprenorphine-naloxone film versus tablets in the management of opioid dependence. *Drug Alcohol Depend*, (2013).

[140] Kapil RP, Cipriano A, Friedman K et al.: Once-Weekly Transdermal Buprenorphine Application Results in Sustained and Consistent Steady-State Plasma Levels. *J. Pain Symptom Manage*, (2012).

[141] Wen W, Lynch SY, Munera C, Swanton R, Ripa SR, Maibach H: Application site adverse events associated with the buprenorphine transdermal system: a pooled analysis. *Expert Opin. Drug Saf.*, (2013).

[142] Davis MP: Buprenorphine in cancer pain. *Supportive care in cancer : official journal of the Multinational Association of Supportive Care in Cancer* 13(11), 878-887 (2005).

[143] Johnson RE, Fudala PJ, Payne R: Buprenorphine: considerations for pain management. *Journal of pain and symptom management* 29(3), 297-326 (2005).

[144] The selection and use of essential medicines. Report of the WHO expert committee, 2005 (including the 14th model list of essential medicines). *World Health Organization technical report series* (933), 1-119, back cover (2006).

[145] Pergolizzi JV, Jr., Mercadante S, Echaburu AV *et al.*: The role of transdermal buprenorphine in the treatment of cancer pain: an expert panel consensus. *Current medical research and opinion* 25(6), 1517-1528 (2009).

[146] Mercadante S, Casuccio A, Tirelli W, Giarratano A: Equipotent doses to switch from high doses of opioids to transdermal buprenorphine.

Supportive care in cancer: official journal of the Multinational Association of Supportive Care in Cancer 17(6), 715-718 (2009).

[147] Mercadante S, Porzio G, Fulfaro F et al.: Switching from transdermal drugs: an observational "N of 1" study of fentanyl and buprenorphine. *Journal of pain and symptom management* 34(5), 532-538 (2007).

[148] Sittl R, Likar R, Nautrup BP: Equipotent doses of transdermal fentanyl and transdermal buprenorphine in patients with cancer and noncancer pain: results of a retrospective cohort study. *Clinical therapeutics* 27(2), 225-237 (2005).

In: Buprenorphine
Editor: Rosalina Bennet
ISBN: 978-1-63321-136-0

Chapter 3

BUPRENORPHINE

K. Vermeylen* and F. Van de Perck
Department of Anesthesia, AZ Turnhout, Turnhout, Belgium

ABSTRACT

Properties, Metabolism and Forms

Buprenorphine is a semi-synthetic derivate of thebaine. [1] Buprenorphine has both analgesic and antihyperalgesic systemic effects [2-4] but the exact mechanism of the different modalities remains unknown. [5] It has three known receptor binding mechanisms. First Buprenorphine is an μ-opioid receptor agonist. Secondly Buprenorphine shows partial agonistic activity at the opioid receptor-like receptor 1 (ORL1)-receptor that induces a pronociceptive effect, for example useful in the treatment of hyperalgesia. Its antagonistic activity at the third receptor, the κ-opioid receptor, might explain the less sedative and psychomimetic effects compared to morphine or fentanyl.

Buprenorphine is metabolised by the liver into norbuprenorphine. The latter is a μ-opioid, δ-opioid and nociception receptor full agonist, as well as a κ-opioid receptor partial agonist. [6, 7] After glucuronidation, both glucuronides are eliminated mainly through excretion into the bile. [8]

* Kris.vermeylen@gmail.com.

Anaesthesiological Clinical Use

A higher-dose sublingual form (up to 2 mg) is indicated for detoxification and long-term replacement therapy in opioid dependency. [9-14] It is also a good alternative to sustained–release opioids such as morphine and oxycodone. [15, 16]. The transdermal form is indicated for the treatment of severe cancer pain and severe non-cancer pain not responding to non-opioids. [17] But also in orthopaedic surgery e.g., in elderly, it is proven an effective tool for pain control [18-20]. The intravenous formulation is used in continuous postoperative pain treatment.

Regional Administration of Buprenorphine

Conflicting results have been published on the efficacy and duration of various opioids (including buprenorphine) in prolonging the duration of local anaesthetics. [21, 22]. The regional use of buprenorphine has been described in neuraxial [23] and peripheral blocks as adjuvants. [21, 22]. Local buprenorphine application, e.g., to the stellate ganglion, is also described in chronical pain management. [24]

Other Clinical Use

Buprenorphine can be sleep-inducing which can be an advantage when pain is accompanied with sleeplessness. [25] Other clinical indications are pregnancy [26], maxillofacial surgery [27], treatment in non-suicidal self-injury [28], vasectomy surgery [29], and due the euphoria and anxiolytic effects it can be used as an alternative antidepressant in patients with depression due to pain.

Adverse Effects and Contraindications

The adverse effects are similar to those of other opioids. The most important side effect is nausea and vomiting, in particular when initiated at high doses.

Another important side- effect is respiratory depression but due to a relatively long half-life, this depression is characterised by a ceiling effect.

[30] The combination with alcohol and/or benzodiazepines however, can lead to fatal respiratory depression.

A "precipitated withdrawal" is described when buprenorphine is used in persons with a physically dependency for full-agonist opioids, who are not already in withdrawal. [31-33]

Conclusion

Buprenorphine is a common used opioid that provide effective pain relief in cancer and non-cancer patients. As an adjuvant used in regional anesthesia, it is likely to? prolong the peripheral nerve block duration.

INTRODUCTION

Buprenorphine hydrochloride was first launched in the 1980s as an analgesic in a sublingual and an injectable form to treat chronic cancer pain and non-malignant pain which does not respond to non-opioid analgesics. [1]Due to misinterpreted animal data many questions about the clinical use remained.

Properties, Metabolism and Forms

Buprenorphine is a semi-synthetic derivate of thebaine with a relatively long half-life, a 2-phase pKa of 8.42 (μ-agonist) and 9.92 (κ-agonist), and an excellent safety profile. [2] It is one of the most chemically reactive opium alkaloids. Its structure is a typically opioid with the inclusion of a C-7 side chain containing a t-butyl group that confers overall lipophilicity on the molecule determining its pharmacology.

Buprenorphine has analgesic and antihyperalgesic systemic effects [3-5] but the exact mechanism of the different modalities remains unknown. [1] Different mechanisms have been suggested for opioid-induced analgesia and antihyperalgesia. But pure μ-opioid receptor agonists however may also contribute to the induction of hyperalgesia. This hyperalgesia could be caused by either the development of tolerance or opioid-induced hyperalgesia, posing a diagnostically dilemma.

Buprenorphine has three known receptor binding mechanisms. First, it is partial μ-opioid receptor agonist with high affinity, but a low intrinsic activity and a slow dissociation from the receptor. These binding properties are responsible for a lower incidence of respiratory or gastro-intestinal effects in comparison with, the also μ-opioid receptor binding, morphine. The binding is relatively slow in comparison with other opioids but the onset of analgesia is not dissimilar, due to an effective analgesia at relatively low receptor occupancy (5-10%). Together with this slow binding there is also a slow dissociation resulting in a long duration of the analgesic effect. Secondly buprenorphine also shows partial agonistic activity at the opioid receptor-like receptor 1 (ORL1)-receptor that is postulated to induce an antinociceptive effect [6-9]. Thirdly, buprenorphine may have an antagonistic activity at a third receptor, the κ-opioid, which in contrast to other full μ agonists exerts an antihyperalgesic effect. [10]

Buprenorphine is metabolised in the liver into norbuprenorphine. Norbuprenorphine is an μ-opioid, δ-opioid and nociceptive receptor full agonist, as well as a κ-opioid receptor partial agonist.—[6, 7] After glucuronidation, both glucuronides are eliminated mainly through excretion into the bile. [8]

Norbuprenorphine is 40 times less analgesic than buprenorphine. [9]

In patients with severe chronic liver disease such as cirrhosis, CYP3A4 activity may be significantly reduced, and metabolism and clearance of buprenorphine may be altered. [10, 11]

As already explained buprenorphine was first marketed in the 1980s as an analgesic in a sublingual and an injectable form.

Subsequently, a polymer matrix patch system has been added. Such transdermal delivery system (TDS) allows passive transdermal diffusion of medication over a prolonged period, while maintaining a constant therapeutic dose. The physicochemical properties of buprenorphine (low molecular weight, high lipophilicity, and high affinity for, as well as slow dissociation from the μ-opioid receptor) makes it well suited for transdermal delivery [12]. A consequence is however, problems associated with oral drug formulations, such as poor absorption from the gastrointestinal tract, hepatic first-pass metabolism, and low and variable bioavailability, may be avoided. [12]

Different kinds of transdermal patches have been produced, ranging from patches delivering over 96 hours up to 7-days delivering patches. Recently a novel implantable formulation, using a polymer matrix sustained-release technology, has been developed but no full FDA approval was yet provided. In addition to a sublingual tablet form, there is also a sublingual film available in different dosages.

Anesthesiological Clinical Use of Buprenorphine

Buprenorphine was first introduced as an analgesic in the 1980s. Depending on the application form, buprenorphine is indicated for the palliation of moderate to severe, acute or chronic pain with no neurological component, or for perioperative analgesia. [13] The antihyperalgesic effect of Buprenorphine may prevent opioid induced hyperalgesia. Yet in orthopaedic surgery, e.g., in elderly, it is proven to perform an effective management of pain control. [14-16]

Buprenorphine was first introduced in the *sublingual* form. This higher-dose sublingual form (up to 2 mg) was and still is indicated for detoxification and long-term replacement therapy in opioid dependency, comparable with methadone.

It is also a good alternative to sustained–release opioids such as morphine and oxycodone. [17-23].

The *transdermal* form has facilitated the maintenance of constant plasma levels of the drug. This form is therefore mainly indicated for the treatment of severe cancer pain and severe non-cancer pain not responding to non-opioids. [24] In case of insufficient pain relief with transdermal application alone, the sublingual form can be used as breakthrough medication.

The *intravenous* formulation is mainly used in continuous postoperative pain treatment.

The role of buprenorphine on the immune system remains unclear. In animal experiments, buprenorphine does not exert immunosuppressive activity at analgesic doses. [25] This is in contrast to morphine, which has been repeatedly shown to be a strong suppressor of various components of the immune system. [26]

The antagonistic activity of Buprenorphine at the κ-opioid, may be partly responsible for the lack of immunosuppression. [27]

Preclinical data from an animal model of lung colonization by tumor cells injected intravenously, showed decreased NK cell activity and augmented tumor metastases with the use of morphine and fentanyl.

Unlike other opioids, buprenorphine was able to prevent neuroendocrine and immune system alterations [28].

These findings suggest that an adequate treatment of surgical stress-induced immunosuppression with an opioid like buprenorphine, which is devoid of immunosuppressive effects in animal experiments, may also play a protective role against the metastatic diffusion following cancer surgery in patients.

This seems to be particularly relevant for some breast, neck, lung and colorectal cancers for which the presence of low NK activity is predictive of poor outcome [29].

Regional Administration of Buprenorphine

Many studies were published in the 1990s showing conflicting results on the efficacy of various opioids (including buprenorphine) in prolonging the duration of local anaesthetics with a wide range in the duration of analgesia, from 10 to 50 hours. [30, 31]

There are some studies on its use in spinal and epidural anaesthesia in combination with e.g., bupivacaine with a prolongation of the block as the result. [32]. But also in peripheral nerve blocks the use of buprenorphine as an adjuvant is described to prolong block duration. [30]

Its use in the treatment of chronic pain is probably the most known. Ganglion local buprenorphine application which application of buprenorphine to the stellate ganglion proves to be very efficient for the treatment of chronic headache and persistent idiopathic facial pain. [33]

No neural toxicity studies have been performed so far but its clinical use in regional techniques has commonly been reported. [30, 31]

Other Clinical Use

Due to its specific characteristics, buprenorphine is presumed to be a safe drug. It can be sleep-inducing which can be an advantage when pain is accompanied with sleeplessness. [34] Other prototypical opioid side effects are characteristic euphoria and anxiolytic effects. Therefore is it sometimes used as an alternative antidepressant in patients with a depression due to pain or patients with intolerance to conventional thymoleptic antidepressants.

Other clinical indications are in pregnancy [35], in maxillofacial surgery [36], treatment of non-suicidal self-injury [37] and vasectomy surgery [38]

Adverse Effects and Contraindications

The adverse effects associated with the use of buprenorphine are similar to those of other opioids and include: nausea and vomiting, drowsiness, dizziness, headache, memory loss, itchiness, constipation (rare), and orthostatic hypotension.

The Most severe side effect is respiratory depression but due to a relatively long half-life, this depression is characterised by a ceiling effect. [39] In combination with alcohol and/or benzodiazepines in concurrent doses, can lead to fatal respiratory depression.

Patients with severe hepatic impairment should be closely monitored during treatment with buprenorphine, and lower initial doses and careful titration is advisable [45]. However, hepatic impairment seems to have only minor, if any effects on the clinical action, pharmacology and clearance of buprenorphine [46]. As buprenorphine is mainly (80–90%) excreted by the biliary system and enterohepatic recirculation, its elimination is not affected by impaired renal function. Normal doses can therefore be given in patients with renal dysfunction, and buprenorphine pharmacokinetics is not altered with advanced age when renal impairment is common. [47-52]

A "precipitated withdrawal" is described when buprenorphine is used in persons with a physical dependency for full-agonist opioids, not yet in withdrawal. The buprenorphine withdrawal is characterised by an extremely intense form? of opioid withdrawal. This reaction depends on the severity of dependence and time elapsed from the last dose. The blockade effect of buprenorphine also blocks endogenous endorphins from binding receptors that can lead to psychological alterations in mood and mental capacity. Allergic reactions or allergic dermatitis and urine retention are also described. [40-42]

Buprenorphine 'State of the Art'

In 2008 a consensus group of experts agreed that buprenorphine clearly behaves as a full μ-opioid agonist for analgesia in clinical practice. [43] They agreed that buprenorphine has a ceiling effect on respiratory depression and the effect can be reversed by Naloxone. But other questions remained. What about the dose-response curves? What about it efficacy in neuropathic pain? What about equipotency ratios, interactions with immune and hormonal systems, and suitability for patients with impaired renal function?

CONCLUSION

Opioids are very important in the treatment of chronic cancer, cancer and noncancer pain. Buprenorphine is a commonly used opioid that provides effective pain relief in this patient population and may offer a number of advantages over the other opioids. But despite the increasing clinical use of buprenorphine, still questions need to be answered concerning a possible ceiling effect for analgesia, the combination with other opioid agonists and the reversibility of side effects.

As an adjuvant it is used successfully in regional anaesthesia, prolonging the peripheral nerve block duration.

REFERENCES FOR ABSTRACT

[1] Steagall PV, Pelligand L, Giordano T, Auberger C, Sear JW, Luna SP, et al. Pharmacokinetic and pharmacodynamic modelling of intravenous, intramuscular and subcutaneous buprenorphine in conscious cats. *Veterinary anaesthesia and analgesia* 2013 Jan;40(1):83-95.

[2] Williams BA, Murinson BB, Grable BR, Orebaugh SL. Future considerations for pharmacologic adjuvants in single-injection peripheral nerve blocks for patients with diabetes mellitus. *Regional anesthesia and pain medicine* 2009 Sep-Oct;34(5):445-57.

[3] Koppert W, Ihmsen H, Korber N, Wehrfritz A, Sittl R, Schmelz M, et al. Different profiles of buprenorphine-induced analgesia and antihyperalgesia in a human pain model. *Pain* 2005 Nov;118(1-2):15-22.

[4] Simonnet G. Opioids: from analgesia to anti-hyperalgesia? *Pain* 2005 Nov;118(1-2):8-9.

[5] Hans G. Buprenorphine--a review of its role in neuropathic pain. *Journal of opioid management* 2007 Jul-Aug;3(4):195-206.

[6] Huestis MA, Cone EJ, Pirnay SO, Umbricht A, Preston KL. Intravenous buprenorphine and norbuprenorphine pharmacokinetics in humans. *Drug and alcohol dependence* 2013 Aug 1;131(3):258-62.

[7] Luthi G, Blangy V, Eap CB, Ansermot N. Buprenorphine and norbuprenorphine quantification in human plasma by simple protein precipitation and ultra-high performance liquid chromatography tandem mass spectrometry. *Journal of pharmaceutical and biomedical analysis* 2013 Apr 15;77:1-8.

[8] Regina KJ, Kharasch ED. High-sensitivity analysis of buprenorphine, norbuprenorphine, buprenorphine glucuronide, and norbuprenorphine glucuronide in plasma and urine by liquid chromatography-mass spectrometry. *Journal of chromatography B, Analytical technologies in the biomedical and life sciences* 2013 Nov 15;939:23-31.

[9] Esses JL, Rosman J, Do LT, Schweitzer P, Hanon S. Successful transition to buprenorphine in a patient with methadone-induced torsades de pointes. *Journal of interventional cardiac electrophysiology : an international journal of arrhythmias and pacing* 2008 Nov;23(2):117-9.

[10] Jones HE, Johnson RE, O'Grady KE, Jasinski DR, Tuten M, Milio L. Dosing adjustments in postpartum patients maintained on buprenorphine or methadone. *Journal of addiction medicine* 2008 Jun;2(2):103-7.

[11] Winstock AR, Lea T, Sheridan J. Patients' help-seeking behaviours for health problems associated with methadone and buprenorphine treatment. *Drug and alcohol review* 2008 Jul;27(4):393-7.

[12] Soyka M, Lieb M, Kagerer S, Zingg C, Koller G, Lehnert P, et al. Cognitive functioning during methadone and buprenorphine treatment: results of a randomized clinical trial. *Journal of clinical psychopharmacology* 2008 Dec;28(6):699-703.

[13] Neumann AM, Blondell RD, Jaanimagi U, Giambrone AK, Homish GG, Lozano JR, et al. A preliminary study comparing methadone and buprenorphine in patients with chronic pain and coexistent opioid addiction. *Journal of addictive diseases* 2013;32(1):68-78.

[14] Havnes IA, Clausen T, Middelthon AL. 'Diversion' of methadone or buprenorphine: 'harm' versus 'helping'. *Harm reduction journal* 2013 Oct 16;10(1):24.

[15] Calderon R, Copenhaver D. Buprenorphine for chronic pain. *Journal of pain & palliative care pharmacotherapy* 2013 Dec;27(4):402-5.

[16] Sharma S, Balireddy RK, Vorenkamp KE, Durieux ME. Beyond opioid patient-controlled analgesia: a systematic review of analgesia after major spine surgery. *Regional anesthesia and pain medicine* 2012 Jan-Feb;37(1):79-98.

[17] Poulain P, Denier W, Douma J, Hoerauf K, Samija M, Sopata M, et al. Efficacy and safety of transdermal buprenorphine: a randomized, placebo-controlled trial in 289 patients with severe cancer pain. *Journal of pain and symptom management* 2008 Aug;36(2):117-25.

[18] Barutell C, Camba A, Gonzalez-Escalada JR, Rodriguez M. High dose transdermal buprenorphine for moderate to severe pain in spanish pain centres--a retrospective multicenter safety and efficacy study. *Pain*

practice: the official journal of World Institute of Pain 2008 Sep-Oct;8(5):355-61.

[19] Likar R, Vadlau EM, Breschan C, Kager I, Korak-Leiter M, Ziervogel G. Comparable analgesic efficacy of transdermal buprenorphine in patients over and under 65 years of age. *The Clinical journal of pain* 2008 Jul-Aug;24(6):536-43.

[20] Krotscheck U, Boothe DM, Little AA. Pharmacokinetics of buprenorphine following intravenous administration in dogs. *American journal of veterinary researc*h 2008 Jun;69(6):722-7.

[21] Viel EJ, Cuvillon P, Eledjam JJ. Opioid and local anesthetic combination for brachial plexus block to provide postoperative analgesia. *Regional anesthesia and pain medicine* 2002 May-Jun;27(3):336.

[22] Viel EJ, Eledjam JJ, De La Coussaye JE, D'Athis F. Brachial plexus block with opioids for postoperative pain relief: comparison between buprenorphine and morphine. *Regional anesthesia* 1989 Nov-Dec;14(6):274-8.

[23] Kanamori M, Ohmori K, Yasuda T, Miaki K, Matsui H, Satone T. Postoperative enteroparesis by patient-controlled analgesia combined with continuous epidural block for patients after posterior lumbar surgery. *Journal of spinal disorders* 2000 Jun;13(3):242-6.

[24] Harris CL, Hamid B, Rosenquist RW, Schultz-Stubner SH. Ganglionic local opioid application (GLOA) for treatment of chronic headache and facial pain. *Regional anesthesia and pain medicine* 2006 Sep-Oct;31(5):460-2.

[25] Hunt JR, Grint NJ, Taylor PM, Murrell JC. Sedative and analgesic effects of buprenorphine, combined with either acepromazine or dexmedetomidine, for premedication prior to elective surgery in cats and dogs. *Veterinary anaesthesia and analgesia* 2013 May;40(3):297-307.

[26] Newman RG, Gevertz SG. Comment on "a comparison of buprenorphine + naloxone to buprenorphine and methadone in the treatment of opioid dependence during pregnancy: maternal and neonatal outcomes". *Substance abuse : research and treatment* 2013;7:107-8.

[27] Wasson M, Beirne OR. Buprenorphine therapy: an increasing challenge in oral and maxillofacial surgery. *Oral surgery, oral medicine, oral pathology and oral radiology* 2013 Aug;116(2):142-6.

[28] Norelli LJ, Smith HS, Sher L, Blackwood TA. Buprenorphine in the treatment of non-suicidal self-injury: a case series and discussion of the

literature. *International journal of adolescent medicine and health* 2013;25(3):323-30.

[29] Wright-Williams S, Flecknell PA, Roughan JV. Comparative effects of vasectomy surgery and buprenorphine treatment on faecal corticosterone concentrations and behaviour assessed by manual and automated analysis methods in C57 and C3H mice. *PloS one* 2013;8(9):e75948.

[30] Megarbane B, Alhaddad H. P-glycoprotein should be considered as an additional factor contributing to opioid-induced respiratory depression in paediatrics: the buprenorphine example. *British journal of anaesthesia* 2013 May;110(5):842.

[31] Boggs CL, Ripple MG, Ali Z, Brassell M, Levine B, Jufer-Phipps R, et al. Anaphylaxis after the injection of buprenorphine. *Journal of forensic sciences* 2013 Sep;58(5):1381-3.

[32] Edwards RT, McCormick-Deaton C, Hosanagar A. Acute urinary retention secondary to buprenorphine administration. *The American journal of emergency medicine* 2014 Jan;32(1):109 e1-2.

[33] Huilaja L, Riekki R, Immonen A, Tasanen K. Allergic Contact Dermatitis from Buprenorphine and Oral Tolerance to Other Opioid Derivatives in Three Patients. *Dermatology* 2013 Nov 23.

References

[1] Hans G. Buprenorphine--a review of its role in neuropathic pain. *Journal of opioid management* 2007 Jul-Aug;3(4):195-206.

[2] Steagall PV, Pelligand L, Giordano T, Auberger C, Sear JW, Luna SP, et al. Pharmacokinetic and pharmacodynamic modelling of intravenous, intramuscular and subcutaneous buprenorphine in conscious cats. *Veterinary anaesthesia and analgesia* 2013 Jan;40(1):83-95.

[3] Williams BA, Murinson BB, Grable BR, Orebaugh SL. Future considerations for pharmacologic adjuvants in single-injection peripheral nerve blocks for patients with diabetes mellitus. *Regional anesthesia and pain medicine* 2009 Sep-Oct;34(5):445-57.

[4] Koppert W, Ihmsen H, Korber N, Wehrfritz A, Sittl R, Schmelz M, et al. Different profiles of buprenorphine-induced analgesia and antihyperalgesia in a human pain model. *Pain* 2005 Nov;118(1-2):15-22.

[5] Simonnet G. Opioids: from analgesia to anti-hyperalgesia? *Pain* 2005 Nov;118(1-2):8-9.

[6] Huestis MA, Cone EJ, Pirnay SO, Umbricht A, Preston KL. Intravenous buprenorphine and norbuprenorphine pharmacokinetics in humans. *Drug and alcohol dependence* 2013 Aug 1;131(3):258-62.

[7] Luthi G, Blangy V, Eap CB, Ansermot N. Buprenorphine and norbuprenorphine quantification in human plasma by simple protein precipitation and ultra-high performance liquid chromatography tandem mass spectrometry. *Journal of pharmaceutical and biomedical analysis* 2013 Apr 15;77:1-8.

[8] Regina KJ, Kharasch ED. High-sensitivity analysis of buprenorphine, norbuprenorphine, buprenorphine glucuronide, and norbuprenorphine glucuronide in plasma and urine by liquid chromatography-mass spectrometry. *Journal of chromatography B, Analytical technologies in the biomedical and life sciences* 2013 Nov 15;939:23-31.

[9] Hand CW, Baldwin D, Moore RA, Allen MC, McQuay HJ. Radioimmunoassay of buprenorphine with iodine label: analysis of buprenorphine and metabolites in human plasma. *Annals of clinical biochemistry* 1986 Jan;23 (Pt 1):47-53.

[10] Hand CW, Ryan KE, Dutt SK, Moore RA, O'Connor J, Talbot D, et al. Radioimmunoassay of buprenorphine in urine: studies in patients and in a drug clinic. *Journal of analytical toxicology* 1989 Mar-Apr;13(2):100-4.

[11] Tegeder I, Lotsch J, Geisslinger G. Pharmacokinetics of opioids in liver disease. *Clinical pharmacokinetics* 1999 Jul;37(1):17-40.

[12] Hans G, Robert D. Transdermal buprenorphine - a critical appraisal of its role in pain management. *Journal of pain research* 2009;2:117-34.

[13] Calderon R, Copenhaver D. Buprenorphine for chronic pain. *Journal of pain & palliative care pharmacotherapy* 2013 Dec;27(4):402-5.

[14] Barutell C, Camba A, Gonzalez-Escalada JR, Rodriguez M. High dose transdermal buprenorphine for moderate to severe pain in spanish pain centres--a retrospective multicenter safety and efficacy study. *Pain practice: the official journal of World Institute of Pain* 2008 Sep-Oct;8(5):355-61.

[15] Likar R, Vadlau EM, Breschan C, Kager I, Korak-Leiter M, Ziervogel G. Comparable analgesic efficacy of transdermal buprenorphine in patients over and under 65 years of age. *The Clinical journal of pain* 2008 Jul-Aug;24(6):536-43.

[16] Krotscheck U, Boothe DM, Little AA. Pharmacokinetics of buprenorphine following intravenous administration in dogs. *American journal of veterinary research* 2008 Jun;69(6):722-7.

[17] Sharma S, Balireddy RK, Vorenkamp KE, Durieux ME. Beyond opioid patient-controlled analgesia: a systematic review of analgesia after major spine surgery. *Regional anesthesia and pain medicine* 2012 Jan-Feb;37(1):79-98.

[18] Esses JL, Rosman J, Do LT, Schweitzer P, Hanon S. Successful transition to buprenorphine in a patient with methadone-induced torsades de pointes. *Journal of interventional cardiac electrophysiology : an international journal of arrhythmias and pacing* 2008 Nov;23(2):117-9.

[19] Jones HE, Johnson RE, O'Grady KE, Jasinski DR, Tuten M, Milio L. Dosing adjustments in postpartum patients maintained on buprenorphine or methadone. *Journal of addiction medicine* 2008 Jun;2(2):103-7.

[20] Winstock AR, Lea T, Sheridan J. Patients' help-seeking behaviours for health problems associated with methadone and buprenorphine treatment. *Drug and alcohol review* 2008 Jul;27(4):393-7.

[21] Soyka M, Lieb M, Kagerer S, Zingg C, Koller G, Lehnert P, et al. Cognitive functioning during methadone and buprenorphine treatment: results of a randomized clinical trial. *Journal of clinical psychopharmacology* 2008 Dec;28(6):699-703.

[22] Neumann AM, Blondell RD, Jaanimagi U, Giambrone AK, Homish GG, Lozano JR, et al. A preliminary study comparing methadone and buprenorphine in patients with chronic pain and coexistent opioid addiction. *Journal of addictive diseases* 2013;32(1):68-78.

[23] Havnes IA, Clausen T, Middelthon AL. 'Diversion' of methadone or buprenorphine: 'harm' versus 'helping'. *Harm reduction journal* 2013 Oct 16;10(1):24.

[24] Poulain P, Denier W, Douma J, Hoerauf K, Samija M, Sopata M, et al. Efficacy and safety of transdermal buprenorphine: a randomized, placebo-controlled trial in 289 patients with severe cancer pain. *Journal of pain and symptom management* 2008 Aug;36(2):117-25.

[25] Van Loveren H, Gianotten N, Hendriksen CF, Schuurman HJ, Van der Laan JW. Assessment of immunotoxicity of buprenorphine. *Laboratory animals* 1994 Oct;28(4):355-63.

[26] Sacerdote P. Opioids and the immune system. *Palliative medicine* 2006;20 Suppl 1:s9-15.

[27] Evans HC, Easthope SE. Transdermal buprenorphine. *Drugs* 2003;63(19):1999-2010; discussion 1-2.

[28] Franchi S, Panerai AE, Sacerdote P. Buprenorphine ameliorates the effect of surgery on hypothalamus-pituitary-adrenal axis, natural killer cell activity and metastatic colonization in rats in comparison with

morphine or fentanyl treatment. *Brain, behavior, and immunity* 2007 Aug;21(6):767-74.

[29] Fujisawa T, Yamaguchi Y. Autologous tumor killing activity as a prognostic factor in primary resected nonsmall cell carcinoma of the lung. *Cancer* 1997 Feb 1;79(3):474-81.

[30] Viel EJ, Cuvillon P, Eledjam JJ. Opioid and local anesthetic combination for brachial plexus block to provide postoperative analgesia. *Regional anesthesia and pain medicine* 2002 May-Jun;27(3):336.

[31] Viel EJ, Eledjam JJ, De La Coussaye JE, D'Athis F. Brachial plexus block with opioids for postoperative pain relief: comparison between buprenorphine and morphine. *Regional anesthesia* 1989 Nov-Dec;14(6):274-8.

[32] Kanamori M, Ohmori K, Yasuda T, Miaki K, Matsui H, Satone T. Postoperative enteroparesis by patient-controlled analgesia combined with continuous epidural block for patients after posterior lumbar surgery. *Journal of spinal disorders* 2000 Jun;13(3):242-6.

[33] Harris CL, Hamid B, Rosenquist RW, Schultz-Stubner SH. Ganglionic local opioid application (GLOA) for treatment of chronic headache and facial pain. *Regional anesthesia and pain medicine* 2006 Sep-Oct;31(5):460-2.

[34] Hunt JR, Grint NJ, Taylor PM, Murrell JC. Sedative and analgesic effects of buprenorphine, combined with either acepromazine or dexmedetomidine, for premedication prior to elective surgery in cats and dogs. *Veterinary anaesthesia and analgesia* 2013 May;40(3):297-307.

[35] Newman RG, Gevertz SG. Comment on "a comparison of buprenorphine + naloxone to buprenorphine and methadone in the treatment of opioid dependence during pregnancy: maternal and neonatal outcomes". *Substance abuse : research and treatment* 2013;7:107-8.

[36] Wasson M, Beirne OR. Buprenorphine therapy: an increasing challenge in oral and maxillofacial surgery. *Oral surgery, oral medicine, oral pathology and oral radiology* 2013 Aug;116(2):142-6.

[37] Norelli LJ, Smith HS, Sher L, Blackwood TA. Buprenorphine in the treatment of non-suicidal self-injury: a case series and discussion of the literature. *International journal of adolescent medicine and health* 2013;25(3):323-30.

[38] Wright-Williams S, Flecknell PA, Roughan JV. Comparative effects of vasectomy surgery and buprenorphine treatment on faecal corticosterone

concentrations and behaviour assessed by manual and automated analysis methods in C57 and C3H mice. *PloS one* 2013;8(9):e75948.
[39] Megarbane B, Alhaddad H. P-glycoprotein should be considered as an additional factor contributing to opioid-induced respiratory depression in paediatrics: the buprenorphine example. *British journal of anaesthesia* 2013 May;110(5):842.
[40] Boggs CL, Ripple MG, Ali Z, Brassell M, Levine B, Jufer-Phipps R, et al. Anaphylaxis after the injection of buprenorphine. *Journal of forensic sciences* 2013 Sep;58(5):1381-3.
[41] Edwards RT, McCormick-Deaton C, Hosanagar A. Acute urinary retention secondary to buprenorphine administration. *The American journal of emergency medicine* 2014 Jan;32(1):109 e1-2.
[42] Huilaja L, Riekki R, Immonen A, Tasanen K. Allergic Contact Dermatitis from Buprenorphine and Oral Tolerance to Other Opioid Derivatives in Three Patients. *Dermatology* 2013 Nov 23.
[43] Pergolizzi J, Boger RH, Budd K, Dahan A, Erdine S, Hans G, et al. Opioids and the management of chronic severe pain in the elderly: consensus statement of an International Expert Panel with focus on the six clinically most often used World Health Organization Step III opioids (buprenorphine, fentanyl, hydromorphone, methadone, morphine, oxycodone). *Pain practice: the official journal of World Institute of Pain* 2008 Jul-Aug;8(4):287-313.

In: Buprenorphine
Editor: Rosalina Bennet
ISBN: 978-1-63321-136-0

Chapter 4

The Application of Buprenorphine in Acute and Chronic Pancreatitis

Wenbo Meng[1,2], Bo Li[2], Yan Li[3], Shaozhen Rui[2], Wence Zhou[2] and Xun Li[2*]
[1]Special Minimally Invasive Surgery, the First Hospital of Lanzhou University, Gansu, China
[2]The Second Department of General Surgery, the First Hospital of Lanzhou University, Hepatopancreatobiliary Surgery Institute of Gansu Province, Clinical Medical College Cancer Center of Lanzhou University, Gansu, China
[3]Department of Immunology, Cleveland Clinic, Cleveland, OH, US

Abstract

Pancreatitis is an inflammation of the pancreas. The most common causes are alcohol consumption and gallstone related. Interestingly, pancreatitis is the most incidence observed in patients following abdominal surgery. The most frequently symptoms of pancreatitis are

* Corresponding author: Xun Li, MD, PhD; Professor of Surgery; The Second Department of General Surgery, the First Hospital of Lanzhou University, Hepatopancreatobiliary Surgery Institute of Gansu Province, Clinical Medical College Cancer Center of Lanzhou University, Lanzhou 730000, Gansu, China. Phone: +86931 8356821; Fax: +86931 8622275; E-mail: drlixun@163.com.

severe abdominal pain, nausea and vomiting. Heart and respiratory function may also be affected. How to reasonably choose a safe, effective and low-dependent analgesic is a big problem faced by the doctors. Analgesics will not affect the recovery of the disease if the patients have chronic or acute inflammation, however it will release the symptoms and make the patients more comfortable. In general, more than one type of analgesics are used in treating pancreatitis, such as acetaminophen, non-steroidal anti-inflammatory drug and opioid etc., which is greatly controversial in clinical application because of the side effects such as ulcers associated with their use. In addition, some studies have shown that the use of opioid may conceal the changes of the disease and because their spasmogenic effects will increase the patients' ache, this in turn increases the sphincter pressure of oddi in abdominal cavity. The biliary tract pressure increase seems to be related with dosage and plasma concentration of opioid and seems to be apparently regulated by the Mu (μ) receptor.

There is a subclass of opioid drug called buprenorphine hydrochloride, along with its relatively outstanding pharmacologic character to be gradually known. buprenorphine can be used as substitute for the drug dolantin in treating the abdominal ache associated with acute and chronic pancreatitis. The use of burprenorphine can be an alternative choice to treat the aching of acute pancreatitis which has less side effects. Compared with other analgesia plans, buprenorphine can reduce analgesia metering needed, and which has no obvious differences in the risk of both the appearances of pancreatitis complication and clinical adverse events. According to the current clinical studies, buprenorphine is the suitable choice for treating the aching of acute pancreatitis, and compared with other analgesia drugs that are not belonging to opioid category. Currently for acute paroxysm associated with chronic pancreatitis, the common suggestions for treatment do not provide enough analgesia effect. Therefore the German Guide suggest the use of dolantin, buprenorphine and procaine administered intravenously as a treatment plan for the abdominal pain resulting from pancreatitis. It is very difficult to control the intractable aching of chronic pancreatitis, but fortunately, it has been reported that buprenorphine is very effective in alleviating the pain that is felt by the patients with chronic pancreatitis. The use of buprenorphine is a simple, safe and effective way compared with current drugs used in treating abdominal ache as a result of pancreatitis.

Abdominal pain is the most common symptom of acute and chronic pancreatitis [1-3], and analgesia treatment is the primary goal of early pancreatitis treatment. The pain always breaks out acutely, reaches the maximum strength after 10-30 minutes, and lasts for several hours without remission [4-5]. In the past dozen years, several analgesia treatments have been recommended in treating acute pancreatitis. Although there is no prospective study to prove its curative effects, intravenous injection of procaine hydrochloride is recommended to relieve the pain of acute pancreatitis [4-7]. In the German Treatment Consensus, procaine is the first choice to treat patients with acute chronic pancreatitis, but there are still some clinicians who prefer derivatives of the opioid category, like dolantin and buprenorphine, and use them as the first choice for basic treatment of analgesia in acute pancreatitis [7-8]. Buprenorphin hydrochloride is the semi-synthetic derivative of the baine category. Buprenorphine possesses the opiate-receptor stimulant and antagonist activities [9]. Compared with morphine, buprenorphine has the characteristics of great analgesic strength, light side-effects of respiratory depression and constipation etc., and low drug dependence [3]. At present, buprenorphine is deeply studied and widely applied in clinical analgesia and rehabilitation treatment.

1. PHARMACODYNAMICS

In vitro, low dosages of buprenorphine shows opiate-receptor stimulant activity, but high dosages appear to function as opiate-receptor antagonists. As a result, in many animal models, the buprenorphine's antalgic dose-effect curve has an inverse U shape, known as the "capping effect [10]. Once the drug dosage reaches a certain blood concentration, the effects will not increase with the dosage, but remain at a certain level and have a higher security [11]. The analgesia effect of buprenorphine is mainly the interactive result between it and μ receptor, and buprenorphine binds with δ receptor to show self-restraint (analgesia activity decline) in high dosage. When μ and κreceptors combine with other opiate stimulants like morphine, buprenorphine shows antagonistic activity, which is the reason using for morphine and meperidine detoxicate. The receptor binding feature of buprenorphine determines that it has a longer analgesia time of duration [12-14], over 6-8h clinically, and 10h in operation. Buprenorphine brings about effects 30-60 minutes after injection, 15-40 minutes after sublingual administration, and reaches its peak after 2 hours. The analgesia effects can last for 5-8 days. The bioavailability is about 55%, the plasma protein binding rate is 96%, and t1/2 is 2-3 hours. The metabolism mainly takes place in liver, and the excretion happens through the gallbladder. It is excreted through feces in its original shape, partially in the kidneys after N-dealkylation, in the liver, and through the blood-brain and placental barriers [15-16].

2. THE EFFECTS OF TREATING PANCREATITIS COMPARED WITH OTHER ANALGESIA DRUGS

The clinical manifestations of acute pancreatitis are quite different. The mild case shows clinical self-confinement, but the severe case has an extremely dangerous prognosis with a fatality rate of 24.14% [17]. Abdominal pain is the major manifestation of acute pancreatitis, and most patients have sudden onset after a full meal or drink. Furthermore, the degrees of pain are quite different, with mild cases reporting dull pain in the upper abdomen and severe cases having eliema and boring pain and lancinated pain (the more severe the lesion, the more acute the pain). To relieve the pain is one of the basic treatments of acute pancreatitis, meanwhile, the abdominal pain is accompanied by nausea, emesis and fever. According to N02A dissection therapeutical chemistry ATC coding (ATC classification), opioids can be classified into: agonist (egmorphine, hydromorphoe, fentanyl), partial agonist (buprenorphine), agonist-antagonist (pentazocine), and opioid antagonist (naloxone) [3]. The opioids are commonly used to control the pain of acute pancreatitis. In order to assess the clinical safety and effectiveness of opioids, the recent system evaluation includes five randomized controlled trials (RCT) and altogether 227 persons (age range 23-76, 65% male), using intravenous and intramuscular injection of buprenorphine, intramuscular injection of pethidine, intravenous injection of pentazocine, the fentanyl transdermal patch and subcutaneously administering morphine, to assess the treating of pain in acute pancreatitis [3]. One of the RCTs shows that intravenous injection of analginum and subcutaneous injection of morphine do not remarkably reduce the patients' pain strength (RR 0.50, 95% CI is 0.19-1.33) [18]. The three studies comparing the analgesia treatment of opioids with non-opioids shows that the number of patients who need extra analgesia drugs obviously declines (RR 0.53, 95% CI is 0.30-0.93). [18-20] For those who use buprenorphine and pethidine as auxiliary analgesia medicine, the increase in numbers of patients who need more analgesia drugs has no significant difference (RR 0.82, 95%CI is 0.61-1.10).[21]. Moreover, the complications in pancreatitis and investigational products have no significant difference. Therefore, compared with other analgesia plans, opioids are the proper choice for treating the pain of acute pancreatitis, and they can reduce the dosage of extra analgesia drugs, at the same time. Compared with other analgesia drugs, the incidence rate of complication of pancreatitis with opioids has no significant difference [22].

The several published studies of using buprenorphine to treat severe pain, like postoperative analgesia, conclude that buprenoephine can effectively relieve pain without severe side effects. Buprenorphine is recommended to treat the pain of acute pancreatitis and acute attack of chronic pancreatitis, but its relevant compared data is limited.

A prospective double blind (with pethidine) study of using buprenorphine to relieve pain of acute pancreatitis shows that 32 patients with acute pancreatitis were randomly allocated to accept intramuscular injection of buprenorphine (0.3 mg, 17 cases) and pethidine (100mg) and a follow-up analgesia (pethidine, 100mg). Only one patient accepting pethidine and four patients accepting buprenorphine did not need extra pethidine, and there was no patient with respiratory depression throughout clinical observation. As a result, buprenorphine and pethidine may provide similar analgesia effects for patients with acute pancreatitis [21].

In the German Treatment Consensus, procaine is recommended as the first choice for patients with acute attack of chronic pancreatitis, although there is no prospective control study in long-term clinical use to prove that procaine is effective in analgesia of pancreatitis. In this study, the analgesia effects of buprenorphine were dramatically better than those of procaine. Buprenorphine effectively relieved the pain of 18 out of 19 patients (94%). The patients in buprenorphine team needed remarkably less extra analgesic than those accepting procaine (1 to 14 cases, $P<0.0001$) [23].

The procaine hydrochloride (procaine) used intravenously has been recommended to relieve pain of acute pancreatitis for several decades. The Goebell and Singer's report showed that about 100 cases of patients had no major side effects by procaine, but accurate data were not recorded. To assess the curative effects and side effects of buprenorphine and procaine toward the patients with acute pancreatitis, 40 patients (average age 50, 23 males) with acute pancreatitis and acute attack of chronic pancreatitis, prospectively, randomly accepted buprenoephine or procaine in continuous intravenous injection. The extra analgesic was added according to the need. The pain score was used in visual analogue scale. The results showed that the patients accepting buprenorphine had a remarkably reduced the need for extra analgesic (1 vs 14 patients, $P<0.0001$) [24-25]. The pain score of patients in buprenorphine team was remarkably lower than that of patients in procaine team ($P<0.05$). The pain score remarkably reduced in the first two days of using buprenorphine more obviously: the first day, 55 to 25, P<0.0001; the second day, 62 to 40, P=0.005. The intravenous injection of buprenorphine is more effective than that of procaine in relieving pain of acute pancreatitis [26].

There seem to be potential dangers for patients who use morphine and derivates of opioids to treat acute pancreatitis, because it will make sphincter of Oddi (SO) contract. Therefore, several research groups investigated the effects of derivates of opioids toward males by measuring pressure of SO, and they discovered that buprenorphine would not cause the contract of SO. The influences of buprenorphine toward the acute experiment of pancreatitis (induced by 3% sodium taurocholate) showed that buprenorphine could obviously reduce the pain but not disturb the process of pancreatitis [27-28].

The main side effects of buprenorphine are drowsiness, dizziness, vomiting and reducing appetite. Through close clinical monitoring, including clinical observation, pulse oxygen and daily blood gas analysis, relevant studies showed no statistically significant difference between treatment with procaine and that with buprenorphine in treating patients' ventilatory dependence [29-34].

The sedation rate was high in the buprenorphine group, and it affected the feeling of pain as well as pain score. If the sedation rate was lowered, the patients who felt pain would benefit, because it would strengthen analgesia effects and the extra analgesic would be reduced. Procaine hydrochloride restrained phospholipase A2, and this was considered a beneficial clinical process for acute pancreatitis. However, a control study showed that this could not be used in the human body. In this study, one patient died during treatment of acute necrotizing pancreatitis by procaine, but there were no deaths in the buprenorphine group. The lengths of hospital stays were 12 days (for buprenorphine) and 14 days (for procaine). Because of ventilatory dependence rates, the adult respiratory distress syndrome happened (1 to 2 cases) [35]. In a word, the continuous intravenous injection of buprenoephine is the more effective treatment measure to relieve the pain than that of procaine.

Therefore, buprenorphine is the proper choice of treating the pain of acute pancreatitis. Compared with other not-opioid analgesic, buprenorphine can reduce analgesia needed. In addition, to manage the intractable pain of chronic pancreatitis is difficult. It is reported that by respectively giving the patients buprenorphine mixture (0.3 mg) and blood (10-15 ml) into epidural space, it took 6 months to relieve the patients' pain [36]. The epidural injection of buprenorphine is an easy, safe and effective way to relieve the pain of chronic pancreatitis.

3. THE APPLICATIONS OF BUPRENORPHINE IN SPECIFIC PATIENTS

The complications with the respiratory system in patients with acute pancreatitis are quite common, and most of patients with acute pancreatitis have respiratory insufficiency manifestation of various degrees. The lesions in the respiratory system as a result of acute pancreatitis will bring difficulty to treatment, and is one of the main reasons of early death of acute pancreatitis.

3.1. The Pathologic Changes

The main pathological manifestations in the lungs of patients with severe acute pancreatitis are pulmonary alveoli, interstitial edema, tiny pulmonary atelectasis, bleeding of pulmonary alveoli, and so on. The lesions in the respiratory system caused by acute pancreatitis may be related to the following factors: 1) Aeration declines, the proportion of aeration and blood flow is imbalanced 2) The effects of pancreatin and its degradation product, and bioactive peptide and 3) The complement system is activated, the alexin-mediated neutrophils gather and deposit in pulmonary alveoli blood vessel and further induce acute respiratory distress syndrome (ARDS) [37-41].

3.2. The Clinical Manifestations

The lesions in the respiratory system caused by acute pancreatitis may be divided into three types according to their development processes and severity degrees: 1) Early respiratory insufficiency with the main feature of hyoxemia, or early occult anoxia 2) Obvious manifestation in lungs, for those who have no improvement in symptoms of acute pancreatitis and in hyoxemia; after having morbidity for 48h, 30%-60% will have obvious pulmonary complications, like pulmonary edema, pleural effusion etc., and dyspnea and rapid pulse will gradually appear for patients. 3) The acute respiratory distress syndrome (ARDS) is the most severe respiratory complication of acute pancreatitis, happening in 15%-20% of the patients with acute pancreatitis, within 2-7 days in the course of disease, or at early stage. The pathological changes in the lungs and the clinical manifestations are similar to ARDS caused by other pathogenesis. The patients have symptoms like accelerated breathing (>35-40 times/min), respiratory distress, and obvious reduction of cyanosis $PaO2(<8.0kPa)$, which cannot be corrected by oxygen uptake. The diffusive dicty-shadow or schistose shadow can be seen in X-ray chest radiography [37-41].

Respiratory depression is the ubiquitous outward effect of opioids and is deepened with increasing dosage. It is fatal when severe respiratory depression occurs because of clinical overdosage, but the respiratory inhibiting effects of opioids are not so similar. Compared with the influences of PCO2 caused by buprenorphine and fentanyl on mice arteries, the results show that PCO2 caused by fentanyl is linearly increasing, but PCO2 by buprenorphine is changing a little. This proved that buprenorphine is an opioid with light respiratory depression and a plateau effect. The respiratory depression caused by buprenorphine in high dosage toward humans also has the same plateau effect as it does in animals. The respiratory inhibiting effects of fentanyl and buprenoephine were compared by a double-blind placebo control with 48 volunteers. In the same analgesia dosage ranges (fentanyl and buprenorphine), the dosage of fentanyl dependently reduced appetite per minute, and breath instability occurred. One volunteer was tested with the highest dosage(500μg/70kg), and long-time breath suspension occurred. For buprenorphine, the similar dosage-dependent respiratory depression occurred at first, however, when dosage was reached, on the contrary of fentanyl, the plateau effect of respiratory depression occurred and kept within 50% of the baseline. If the highest dosage was reached (600μg/70kg), there was no unstable breathing, periodic breathing or breath suspension. Dahall et al. further discussed the effect features of the human respiratory depression and analgesia caused by buprenorphine. Each person of two groups of volunteers (10 persons in each group) accepted buprenorphine 3 and 6μg/kg separately. The results showed that if the dosage increased from 3μg/kg to 6μg/kg, respiratory inhibiting effects had no change but the analgesia effects significantly enhanced. In the dosage range of completely effective analgesia, buprenorphine had plateau effects, but analgesia effects had no plateau effects. As a result, It is quite safe to use buprenorphine in treating clinical pain [42-43].

The excretory functions of the kidneys generally decrease with the increase in age of elderly patients. The function of the kidneys of patients always gets damaged by hypertension and diabetes. Low renal function can lower the drug metabolism and affect the safety of clinical medication. The active metabolites of opioids, like morphine and codeine, forming in liver conduct analgesia treatment on patients with chronic pain and low renal function by clearing away metabolites accumulated within the kidneys with prototype objects and cause severe outward effects. For these patients, the dosage should be considered to be lowered, and the pharmacy interval should be prolonged. Different from the aforementioned drug, the liver metabolites of buprenorphine are mostly excreted through bile and the prototype metabolites through feces, and the medicine does not accumulate for those with low renal function. As a result, buprenorphine is the first choice of analgesia drug for the elderly and the patients with damaged renal function [44].

4. The Pathological Reasons of Treating Pancreatitis with Buprenorphine

During acute pancreatitis, pancreatin secretion is inhibited, so the content of zymogen in acinus increases. The premature excitation of zymogen is considered to play the central role in the pathogenesis of acute pancreatitis. It can furthest reduce the storage content of zymogen, and it will then induce severe acute pancreatitis. The synthesis of inhibitory enzyme or the secretion of stimulant enzyme will both induce the decline of stored zymogen. The opioid exerts different influences on pancreatic secretion, and this depends on the dosage, dose position and whether pancreas stimulants exist. Through an experiment, how opioids influence the pancreas enzymatic synthesis was studied. Four groups of mice: the first group accepted cerulein 25μg/kg, the second group accepted opioid and buprenorphine (BPN, 0.5mg/kg) and the third accepted cerulain and BPN. The drugs dissolved in gelatin/saline and were injected subcutaneously. The fourth group (control group) only got gelatin/saline. The mice were executed 4 hours after dose and the weights of the pancreases were measured, and the contents of amylase and DNA of pancreas acinus were prepared and detected. The synthesis of amylase, trypsin, chymotrypsin and lipase and the secretion of amylase were measured for 2 hours. Compared with the control group, the content of amylase in acinus of mice with pancreatitis increased, in agreement with the decline of the secretion of amylase in the bodies of the mice. Compared with the control group, the synthetic ratios of the total protein and individual enzymes of mice with pancreatitis were remarkably lower. The synthesis of negative-feedback inhibitory enzyme is because of the increase of the stored enzyme within cells, which could explain these findings. In mice with acute pancreatitis, buprenorphine relieved the edema of pancreas. The amylase in acinus of mice with acute pancreatitis was remarkably lower in those treated with buprenorphine than in those not. Because the amylase was lower in mice with acute pancreatitis and treated with buprenorphine, the decline of amylase contents in acinus can only be because of the decline of pancreatin synthesis in that group. As a result, all the findings proved that buprenorphine could adjust the development of AP [45-48].

5. The Whole Body or Local Drug Delivery

The intravenous medications of clinical or animal experiments demonstrate that it is safe and effective to give buprenorphine through intravenous medications. Even when over-dosage of buprenorphine is used, there happens no obvious respiratory depression. There are studies that compared patient controlled analgesia (PCIA) with epidural PCEA for patients through intravenous medications. The study chose 54 elderly patients (<65 age), who were all patients after excision of gall bladder by laparoscope, ASA I-II class and divided them into two groups randomly. The group A accepted intravenous PCIA with the buprenorphine's dosage of 20 mg/ml; The group B accepted epidural PCEA with the buprenorphine's dosage of 5 mg/ml, combining 0.125% of bupivacaine. The results showed that compared with the group that received epidural PCA, the group of intravenous PCA was not easily affected by hypotension and bradycardia, and the haemodynamics stability was higher, because the intravenous PCA excused the operation processes of epidural anesthesia, and the patients felt more satisfied [49].

The continuous intravenous injection of buprenorphine has better analgesia effects than that of procaine. In a German open study, 40 patients with acute or chronic pancreatitis randomly accepted the intravenous injection of buprenorphine 0.3mg and later accepted the intravenous injection of buprenorphine 2.4mg/day (n=19) or the intravenous injection of procaine 2g/day (24-72h). Compared with the buprenrophine group, in the procaine group, a remarkably small patient needed extra analgesic (5.2% to 70%) and reduced from base-line ache score from the first day (-55 to -25) to the second day (-62 to -40) [22].

The correlation function of oral administration of buprenorphine is obvious, thus oral administration has bad effects.

As a result, the randomized controlled trials of comparing different analgesic are of low quality and do not clearly favor analgesics of any specific acute pancreatitis. Buprenorphine has the characteristics of strong pharmacologic action, small molecular weight, appropriate water solubility and higher lipotropy, and is suitable to be made as a transdermal patch. However, there is no study about a buprenorphine patch being used to treat acute pancreatitis, and it is up for further studies in the future.

6. The Side Effects of Buprenorphine

Buprenorphin hydrochloride belongs to high lipophilic-class drug, and it has opiate-receptor stimulant and antagonistic activities. Low dosages of buprenorphine shows activity of opiate receptor stimulant, but in high dosages, it appears to function as an opiate receptor antagonist. Buprenorphine does not cause agitated or uncomfortable feelings, has lower side effects, like respiratory depression or constipation, and smaller medicine dependence potential [49-51].

However, there was a report of pancreatitis caused by buprenoephine. The patient was a 31-year-old female, and she had a history of addiction to heroin and HCV infection, and had already accepted the replacement therapy of buprenoephine, keeping under tongue. There appeared to be bleeding and precordial pain after intravenously injecting 8mg of buprenorphine and a tablet already smashed and dissolved in water. On the second day after being given these, there appeared abdominal pain and an increase of serum amylase and lipase for her. Meanwhile, iconography reminded the diagnosis of acute pancreatitis. Later on, the patient was transferred to the ICU, given acetaminophen and nefopam, and buprenorphine was replaced with adanon. The patient left the hospital with improvements after treatment. This patient was considered to be one with acute pancreatitis induced by the drug, and after searching the AdisBase and MEDLINE, there is no report relevant to buprenorphine-related pancreatitis. The World Health Organization's adverse drug reaction database includes three reports of pancreatitis related to buprenorphine [52].

Buprenorphine is an efficient analgesic to treat pain of the acute and chronic pancreatitis. Unique pharmacological and biochemical properties make buprenorphine relatively safe and relatively flexible in dosage and dosage form usage. So, buprenorphine is likely to become an pain-treatment drug with wide foreground.

ACKNOWLEDGMENTS

We would like to express our deepest gratitude to Professor Kiyohito Tanaka, Department of Gastroenterology, Kyoto Second Red Cross Hospital in Japan, for his excellent guidance, assistance, patience review. E-mail: seijin7705@gmail.com

REFERENCES

[1] Paisley P1, Kinsella J. Pharmacological management of pain in chronic pancreatitis. *Scott Med. J.* 2014; 59(1):71-9.

[2] Poulsen JL1, Olesen SS; Malver LP, Frøkjær JB. et al. Pain and chronic pancreatitis: a complex interplay of multiple mechanisms. *World J. Gastroenterol.* 2013; 19(42): 7282-91.

[3] Basurto OX, Rigau CD, Urrútia G. Opioids for acute pancreatitis pain. *Cochrane Database Syst. Rev.* 2013; 26;7:CD009179.

[4] Lankisch PG, Banks P. Acute pancreatitis. Berlin: Springer-Verlag; 1996.

[5] Banks P. Practice guidelines in acute pancreatitis. *Am. J. Gastroenterol.* 1997; 92:377–86.

[6] Lankisch PG. Acute and chronic pancreatitis. An update on management. *Drugs.* 1984; 28:554– 64.

[7] Baron TH, Morgan DE. Current concepts: acute necrotizing pancreatitis. *N. Engl. J. Med.* 1999; 340:1412– 7.

[8] Mo¨ssner J, Keim V; Niederau C, Bu¨chler M. et al. Guidelines for the treatment of chronic pancreatitis. *Z. Gastroenterol.* 1998; 36:359– 67.

[9] Hanks GW. Opioid analgesics in the management of pain in patients with cancer. A review. Palliat Med. 1987; 1:1–25.

[10] Rance MJ. Animal and molecular pharmacology of mixed agonist-antagonist analgesic drugs. *Br. J. Clin. Pharmacol.* 1979; 7 Suppl 3:281S-286S.

[11] Dahan A, Yassen A; Romberg R, Sarton E, Teppema L. et al. Buprenorphine induces ceiling in respiratory depression but not in analgesia. *Br. J. Anaesth.* 2006; 96(5):627-32.

[12] Downing JW, Leary WP, White ES. Buprenorphine: a new potent long-acting synthetic analgesic. Comparison with morphine. *Br. J. Anaesth.* 1977; 49(3):251-5.

[13] Lutfy K, Cowan A. Buprenorphine: a unique drug with complex pharmacology. *Curr. Neuropharmacol.* 2004; 2(4):395-402.

[14] Lutfy K, Eitan S; Bryant CD, Yang YC. et al. Buprenorphine-induced antinociception is mediated by mu-opioid receptors and compromised by concomitant activation of opioid receptor-like receptors. *J. Neurosci.* 2003 ;23(32):10331-7.

[15] Escher M, Daali Y; Chabert J, Hopfgartner G. et al. Pharmacokinetic and pharmacodynamic properties of buprenorphine after a single intravenous administration in healthy volunteers: a randomized, double-blind, placebo-controlled, crossover study. *Clin. Ther.* 2007; 29(8):1620-31.

[16] Park I, Kim D, Song J. Bupredernn, a new transdermal delivery system of buprenorphine: pharmacokinetic, efficacy and skin irritancy studies. *Pharm. Res.,* 2008; 25(5):1 052—62.

[17] Li GK, Tian FZ; Su YP, Li X. Impact of secondary pancreatic infection on the prognosis of patients with severe acute pancreatitis: an analysis of 60 cases. *Zhongguo Wei Zhong Bing Ji Jiu Yi Xue.* 2004; 16(1): 2-5.

[18] Peiro AM, Martínez J; Martínez E, DeMadaria E, et al. .Efficacy and tolerance of metamizole versus morphine for acute pancreatitis pain. *Pancreatology.* 2008;8 (1):25–9.

[19] Jakobs R, Adamek MU; Von Bubnoff AC, Riemann JF. Buprenorphine or procaine for pain relief in acute pancreatitis. A prospective randomized study. *Scandinavian Journal of Gastroenterology.* 2000; 35(12):1319–23,

[20] Kahl S, Zimmermann S; Pross M, Schulz HU, et al. Procaine hydrochloride fails to relieve pain in patients with acute pancreatitis. *Digestion.* 2004;69(1):5–9.

[21] Blamey SL, Finlay IG, Carter DC, Imrie CW. Analgesia in acute pancreatitis: comparison of buprenorphine and pethidine. *BMJ Clinical Research. 1984*; 288(6429):1494–5,

[22] Jakobs R, Adamek MU; Von Bubnoff AC, Riemann JF. Buprenorphine or procaine for pain relief in acute pancreatitis. A prospective randomized study. *Scandinavian Journal of Gastroenterology* 2000;35(12):1319–23,

[23] Mo¨ssner J, Keim V; Niederau C, Bu¨chler M. et al.. Guidelines for the treatment of chronic pancreatitis. *Z. Gastroenterol* 1998;36:359– 67.

[24] Goebell H, Singer MV. Acute pancreatitis: standards of conservative treatment. In: Beger HG, Bu¨chler M, editors. Acute pancreatitis. Berlin: Springer-Verlag. 1987. p. 259–65.

[25] Glazer G. Early non-operative management of acute pancreatitis. In: Glazer G, Ranson JHC, editors. Acute pancreatitis. Experimental and clinical aspects of pathogenesis and management.London: Baillie`re Tindall. 1988. p. 331–57.

[26] Meng Wb, Yuan J; Zhang C, Bai Z. et al. Parenteral analgesics for pain relief in acute pancreatitis: a systematic review *Pancreatology*. 2013; 13(3):201-6.

[27] Cuer JC, Dapoigny M; Ajmi S, Larpent JL. et al. Effects of buprenorphine on motor activity of the sphincter of Oddi in man. *Eur. J. Clin. Pharmacol*. 1989; 36:203– 4.

[28] Staritz M, Poralla T; Manns M, Meyer Z. Effect of modern analgesic drugs (tramadol, pentazocine, and buprenorphine) on the bile duct sphincter in man. *Gut*. 1986; 27(5):567-9.

[29] Landau CJ, Carr WD; Razzetti AJ, Sessler NE. et al. Buprenorphine transdermal delivery system in adults with persistent noncancer-related pain syndromes who require opioid therapy: a multicenter, 5-week run-in and randomized, double-blind maintenance-of-analgesia study. *Clin. Ther*. 2007; 29(10):2179-93.

[30] Likar R Griessinger N, Sadj ak A Transdermal buprenorphine for treatment of chronic tumor and non tumor pain *Wien Med. Wochenschr*. 2003;153(13.14):3 17-22.

[31] Marbane B, Hreiche R, Pimay S. Does high—dose buprenorphine cause respiratory depression:possible mechanisms and therapeutic consequences *Toxicol. Rev*. 2006;25(2):79-85.

[32] Ilblick NG, Siller M, Sffdhandske T Effects of buprenorphine on body temperature, locomotor activity and cardiovascular function when assessed by telemetric monitoring in rats. *Lab. Anim*. 2008;42(2):1 49—60.

[33] Shafford HL, Schadt JC. Effect of buprenorphine on the cardiovascular and respiratory response to visceral pain in conscious rabbits. *Vet Anaesth Analg*. 2008; 1 8(5):234—5.

[34] Wedam EF, Bigelow GE, Johnson RE QT-Interval Effects of Methadone, Levomethadyl, and Buprenorphine in a Randomized Trial. *Arch. Intern. Med*. 2007;1 67(22):2469—75.

[35] Yoshikawa T, Naruse S; Kitagawa M, Ishiguro H. et al. Effect of a new inhibitor of type II phospholipase A2 on experimental acute pancreatitis in rats. *Pancreas*. 1999; 19(2):193-8.

[36] Desai PM. Pain relief in chronic pancreatitis with epidural buprenorphine injection. *Indian J. Gastroenterol*. 1997; 16(1):12-3.

[37] Otsuki M1, Takeda K; Matsuno S, Kihara Y. et al. Criteria for the diagnosis and severity stratification of acute pancreatitis. *World J. Gastroenterol.* 2006; 19(35):5798-805.

[38] Kota SK1, Krishna SV; Lakhtakia S, Modi KD. Metabolic pancreatitis: Etiopathogenesis and management. *Indian J. Endocrinol. Metab.* 2013; 17(5):799-805.

[39] Elder AS1, Saccone GT, Dixon DL. Lung injury in acute pancreatitis: mechanisms underlying augmented secondary injury. *Pancreatology.* 2012; 12(1):49-56.

[40] Zhou MT1, Chen CS; Chen BC, Zhang QY. et al. Acute lung injury and ARDS in acute pancreatitis: mechanisms and potential intervention. *World J. Gastroenterol.* 2010; 16(17):2094-9.

[41] Rünzi M1, Layer P. Etiology, pathogenesis and pathophysiology of acute pancreatitis *Schweiz Med. Wochenschr.* 1997; 127(20):849-53.

[42] Dahan A Opioid-induced respiratory effects: new data on buprenophine . *Palliat Med.* 2006; 20(Suppl 1): 3-8.

[43] Dahan A, Yassen A, Bijl H. Comparison of the respiratory effects of intravenous buprenophine and fentanyl in humanns and rars. *Br. J. Anaesth.* 2005; 94(6): 825-834.

[44] Boger RH. Renal impairment: a challenge for opioid treatment? The role of buprenorphine. *Palliat Med.* 2006; 20(suppll): 17-23.

[45] Gilliland L, Steer ML. Effects of ethionine on digestive enzyme synthesis and discharge by mouse pancreas. *Am. J. Physiol.* 1980; 239(5):G418-26

[46] Powers RE, Saluja A; Houlihan MJ, Steer ML: Diminished agonist-stimulated inositol triphosphate generation blocks stimulus-secretion coupling in pancreatic acini during dietinduced experimental pancreatitis. *J. Ciin. Invest.* 1986 ;77:1668- 1674.

[47] Koike H, Steer ML, Meldolesi J. Pancreatic effects of ethionine: blockade of exocytosis and appearance of crinophagy and autophagy precede cellular necrosis. *Am. J. Physiol.* 1982; 242(4):G297-307.

[48] Geokas MC, Rinderknecht V, Swanson V, Haverback BJ: The role of elastase in acute haemorrhagic pancreatitis inman. *Lab. Invest.* 1968; 19:235-239.

[49] Nishikawa K, Kimura S, Shimodate Y. A comparison of intravenous ased and epidural based techniques for anesthesia and postoperative analgesia in elderly patients undergoing laparoocopic cholecystectomy. *Anesth. 2007*; 21(1):l-6.

[50] J.W, Lewis. Buprenorphine. *Drug and Alcohol Dependence*. 1985; 14(3-4): 363.

[51] Nancy K Mello, Jack H Mendelson. Bchavioral pharmacology of buprenorphine. *Drug and Alcohol Dependence*. 1985; 14(3-4):283.

[52] Sepulveda S, Dermine H, Mulot A, Villard M, et al. Acute pancreatitis after intravenous buprenorphine misuse in a heroin addict. *Ann Fr Anesth Reanim.* 2004; 23(6):658-663.

In: Buprenorphine
Editor: Rosalina Bennet

ISBN: 978-1-63321-136-0

Chapter 5

SUBSTITUTION MAINTEINANCE TREATMENT OF OPIOID DEPENDENCE WITH BUPRENORPHINE/NALOXONE METHOD AS PREVENTION OF SOCIAL EXCLUDING OF YOUNG PEOPLE: TUZLA MODEL

Mevludin Hasanović*[1,2]*, Izet Pajević*[1,2]*,
Abdurahman Kuldija*[1]*, Amra Delić*[3]*,
***Alija Sutović*[1,2] *and Esmina Avdibegović*[1,2]**

[1]Department of Psychiatry, University Clinical Center Tuzla, Tuzla, Bosnia-Herzegovina
[2]School of Medicine, University of Tuzla, Tuzla, Bosnia-Herzegovina
[3]Primary Health Care Center Tuzla, Tuzla, Bosnia-Herzegovina

ABSTRACT

Aim: To present medical assisted treatment of opiate dependence with substitution medicament Buprenorphine/Naloxone (Suboxone®) in Bosnia and Herzegovina, with which we may prevent social excluding of young individuals who were opiate dependants.

General overview: Until recently there was no solution for long-term and comprehensive treatment of young persons who suffer from opiate dependency. This is not illness that impairs only psychical health of addicts with possible life threatening consequences, but this is serious problem in whole society because of aftereffects that lead young people in social excluding: delinquencies, criminals, violations and imprisonments. In health care institutions there are no capacities for the stationary treatment for longer term, what is necessary for the treatment of drug dependence, and less adequate solution is seating in penal and upbringing institutions, which, besides stigmatizing young protégés, it excludes young addicts from normal social life in addition. The most modern medically assisted method of substitution treatment of opiate dependants with medical substance Buprenorphine/Naloxone (Suboxone®) has been implemented. This medicament with its characteristics offers possibility for out-patient treatment. With this it is possible to achieve prompt and effective results of detoxification and weaning of opiates. Treated opiate dependants become "clear minded", qualified for the all professional and social activities, what improves significantly quality of family and social relationship. With this way the treatment in the institutions can be avoided, therefore it preventing social excluding of young person's treated with this method.

Conclusion: Medical assisted treatment of opiate dependence with Buprenorphine/Naloxone is implementing outpatient program with involvement of close family members who are not drug dependants. It brings back "clear mind" to treated young opiate addicts, it does not stigmatize but it re-socialize and in that way it is preventing social excluding of young opiate dependant persons.

Keywords: Bosnia and Herzegovina, Tuzla Model, Opiate dependence, Substitution therapy, Medical assisted treatment, Buprenorphine /Naloxone, Suboxone®, Social excluding

INTRODUCTION

Even though population perspectives on specific addictive behaviors, such as drinking or drug use, have been extensively studied in many countries, there is very little research on how people in different societies see diverse addictions in relation to each other [1]. In each country of the world today, the emergence of substance abuse and addiction, especially if they have an increasing trend, represents significant health, economic, social and cultural problem, while for Bosnia and Herzegovina, this phenomenon means an additional burden in the long and complicated transition process of recovery after the end of the war in 1995. In the general atmosphere of destruction, social and economic crisis, the inversion of values and illegal drug trafficking, quite expectedly, there was an increase in the number of people who experiment with drugs and increase in the number of addicts [2]. As it is known substance abuse is a serious disease that impairs psychological and physical health of users, often with fatal consequences (HIV, hepatitis B and C, which is common with a death due to an overdose or other life-threatening conditions in which they find themselves addicted looking for psychoactive substances) [3]. This is a problem that society is forced to endure the consequences of addictive behavior, delinquency, criminal activity and violence [4, 5]. Health facilities are not able to provide accommodation stationary for a longer period, which is necessary for the treatment of drug addiction, while correctional institutions and prisons are not an adequate solution to this problem, because in most cases it is only delaying the consequences of addictive behaviors on society and the environment [6].

Therefore, in the Department of Psychiatry of the University Clinical Center Tuzla with consent of Management of the University Clinical Center Tuzla, Tuzla Canton Institution for Health Insurance (ZZOTK) and the Tuzla Canton Ministry of Health, we began the medical assisted substitution maintenance treatment of opiate addicts with the Buprenorphine/Naloxone (Suboxone®), on the 27th July 2009 year, which was developed into a unique concept called "Tuzla model treatment of opiate addiction with Buprenorphine/Naloxone", which is appropriate to the existing social and financial circumstances [7].

After the meeting in the office of Tuzla Canton Health Ministry under the leadership of the Tuzla Canton Health Minister in the presence of: Minister of Internal affairs of Tuzla Canton and his spokesman, Director of the Primary Health Center „Dom zdravlja" Tuzla and his Deputy, Director of the Tuzla Canton Institution for Health Insurance and Medical Director of University Clinical Center Tuzla and representatives of Department of Psychiatry, University Clinical Center Tuzla, it was decided that Buprenorphine/Naloxone can be prescribed only from the licensed specialists of Neuro-psychiatry approved by the Tuzla Canton Health Minister.

This method ensures that young people from the beginning return to a healthy life, and that in the perspective of the community are able to give back much more than it was invested into their treatment, contrary to those patients whose disease, despite high treatment undertaken, ending with permanent disability, inability to go back to their operations, remain incurable and finally cause the death, like lung cancer caused by tobacco smoking [8].

The treatment of heroin addicts cannot be only a job of psychiatrists and the Department of Psychiatry; a complex synchronized and phase-defined actions of all entities in the community should contribute through all three levels of prevention of drug addiction [4, 9].

With this method, we give the arguments that we are able to resist and successfully cope with this past daunting social and medical evilness [10].

We emphasize that all heroin addicts who are in the "Tuzla model treatment of opiate addiction with Buprenorphine/Naloxone", are treated from the team consisted from the two specialists in neuropsychiatry, nurses, psychologist and social worker in the common rooms of the Ward of Social Psychiatry, together with all other inpatients and outpatients during our regular clinical work. This helps to opiate addicts to feel as regular patients without stigma problems, also it helps to other patients to go over their fears of meeting and talking with heroin addicts and their families.

Our Experiences in the Treatment of Opiate Addicts Using Buprenorphine/Naloxone

Department of Psychiatry in the University Clinical Center (UCC) from Tuzla since 2002. year established a close and fruitful international cooperation with the Clinic for addiction "Beröendecentrum" University Hospital in Örebro in Sweden. Through this cooperation we profiled our doctrine, which is based on the experiences and latest developments in the world which are applicable in Sweden. Our two prominent experts in this area stayed in January and February 2005 in the study visit in Örebro at Clinic for addiction, where they acquired theoretical and practical knowledge on the application of buprenorphine in the treatment of opiate addicts. Buprenorphine has been added to the list of essential drugs of the World Health Organization (WHO) in March 2005, and from January 2007 in Croatia, neighbor country of Bosnia and Herzegovina (BH). Regarding our working conditions and lack of possibility to employ new workers for this particular therapeutic work with opiate addicted clients, we decided to start with planning of opiate substitution therapy in the existing rooms with existing medical staff. As in Bosnia and Herzegovina already institutions for treatment of drug addicts and alcoholics had been established separately from Psychiatry Departments, and they established treatment protocol of opiate addicts based on Methadone only, we established model in which we planned to administrate Buprenorphine /Naloxone only.

In the Federation of BH (FBH) Buprenorphine/Naloxone was registered in December 2007 year. Government of the FBH on their 66th session on 19.08.2008 adopted a decision on which the Buprenorphine/Naloxone was included in "A" list of essential medicines, necessary to provide health care within the standards of mandatory health insurance in the FBH. At the Department of Psychiatry in Tuzla, we started with a new method of treatment of opiate addicts from 27.07.2009 year, after the authorized distributor successfully acquired Buprenorphine/Naloxone in their warehouse.

Determined to help addicts and their families, we faced with the lack of regulation and economic problem. Regardless the FBH Government included new medicine in the "A" essential list, Tuzla Canton Government did not prepared a particular Doctrine for distribution of Buprenorphine/Naloxone. As we had patients who wanted to start with treatment of their opiate dependency, we suggested them to start applying substitution maintenance therapy of opiate addicts with these new drugs, if they agree to buy medicine for their own money. Also we suggested them to keep their receipts and to demand allowance after they buy and use Buprenorphine/Naloxone, because Cantonal Institution for Health Insurance was not redeemed this medication for a list of essential medicines, and they did not prescribe a special doctrine that the medication would be prescribed by the legislation.

Thanks to unquestionable consent of concerned addict and their families, we began the gradual practical clinical application of this drug in the treatment. Because of our particular conditions, the Buprenorphine/Naloxone included according our own original doctrine, established under the circumstances respecting the real scope of life of drug addicts, our working conditions at the Department in strict adherence to medical and legal principles.

The doctrine is based on the following principles:

1. Maximum control of medication
2. Elimination of all forms of addictive behavior
3. Partner involvement of family members of addicts who are addicted to the psycho active substance (PAS)
4. Reliable coordination with pharmacy
5. Detection and integrated interdisciplinary treatment of infections of HIV, hepatitis B and C
6. Detection and integrated treatment of dual diagnosis

7. Discovering the trials and prescribed penal measures, and assisting in serving a quality behavior in court action that is carried out in a penal institution
8. Fighting Stigma and successful rehabilitation and resocialization

The ultimate goal is to bring a drug addict to a degree that is removed from the substitution and continue life as a healthy, rehabilitated and re-socialized [11], in other words the ultimate goal is to enable an individual to achieve lasting abstinence without substitution, to become rehabilitated and resocialized to continue more healthful lifestyle going back to the point where they stopped their regular development, and to help them to find their continuity of human development and to become useful community members to the rest of their lives [11].

Maximum Control of Medication

Since we began to administer Buprenorphine/Naloxone, before the Cantonal Institution for Health Insurance adopted the doctrine of it's administration, the families of the addicts were paid drugs to 17.02.2010 when the Cantonal Institution for Health Insurance in agreement with the Tuzla Canton Minister of Health and the Management of the University Clinical Center Tuzla, and Department of Psychiatry, accepted and made official very efficient newly established model that we developed on the model of the most modern theoretical and practical achievements [8].

After a detailed medical evaluation and psychosocial preparation of an addict, along with establishing collaboration with her/his parents and/or spouse or significant other that is not addicted, a council of specialists that lead the expert team of our Department decide of the introduction of opiate addict to treatment program with Buprenorphine/Naloxone. If the members of the consilium find no contraindications for this treatment option, an addict and her/his partner in the treatment who is not addicted (parent, spouse or significant other) sign the contract with consilium, which regulates that Suboxone pills will be taken regularly, in proper dosage, in a prescribed manner, and that it won't be misused or alienated any of the tablet with an awareness of the criminal responsibility for interrupting treatment and illegal distribution of pills.

Thereafter an addict and her/his treatment partner sign an informed consent to medical conditions of treatment, which regulates the strict abstinence of illegal psychoactive substances, as well as of alcohol and benzodiazepines, which in case of its simultaneous use represent a fatal complication of the treatment with Buprenorphine/Naloxone. The informed consent is also signed by the president of the consilium with a guarantee for regularity of drug administration according to the doctrine. The contract created in this way represents an official document signed by three parties about obligations and rights of drug addict, her/his family/significant other, and professionals as service providers. All data is kept in the system and stored within the medical records.

Prescriptions are prescribed in two copies only by two specialists psychiatrists from the Department of Psychiatry (currently Dr. A. Kuldija and Prof. M. Hasanović), authorized by the Ministry for Health of Tuzla Canton, Institute for Health Insurance of Tuzla Canton (ZZO TK), University Clinical Center Tuzla and Department for Psychiatry, who have their own coded stamps entered in the upper right corner of the prescription. Prescriptions are verified by the doctor with his signature and stamp on its back too. Only one pharmacy in Tuzla Canton is authorized for Buprenorphine/Naloxone procurement, where the signatures and signed copies of an informed consent of addicts and their treatment partners are being deposited. The manager and the pharmacy staff closely cooperate with specialists in case of any ambiguities, inconsistencies or doubts about possible misuse of prescriptions. According to the doctrine adopted in Tuzla Canton, the Institute of Health

Insurance of Tuzla Canton provides up to 8 mg of Suboxone daily per addict for free, while the rest of dosage, if needed (daily dose over 8 mg) is self-paid. The costs of Buprenorphine/Naloxone purchase from 27 July 2009 to 17 February 2010, in a period prior to doctrine guidelines development, were reimbursed (part of the cost up to 8 mg) by the cantonal health system.

After signing the informed consent, addicts begin treatment with a gradual introduction, controlling withdrawal for at least 24 hours after the last intake of opiate, starting with 4 mg sublingually. The dose is titrated during an emergency period of no longer than four days. On the fourth day most addicts are generally stable, clear-minded, doing well and continue on a steady dose taken on the 4th day. In the following one-month period the patient must visit the doctor on a limited basis - once a week- when urine screening is used and, if negative, the new prescription is prescribed. From then, the patient is assessed every 28 days and urine screening is mandatory (opiates, BZD and other psychoactive substances).

Elimination of All Forms of Addictive Behavior

The patients are asked to stop taking all PAS (including benzodiazepines and alcohol) due to their possible fatal complications. Treatment must not be initiated if the patient is positive to substances other than opiate. All of them are obliged to wait until the urine test becomes negative on particular PAS except on opiate. When it becomes negative the further procedure of initiation of treatment may continue to its realization.

If the addict is tobacco/cigarettes smoker, then we start motivational interview to help him or her to become motivated to cease tobacco/cigarette smoking. They are offered substitution therapy with Niccorette® chewing gum and/or sticking plasters, which contribute to reduction of overall addictive behavior and the promotion of healthy lifestyle.

Partner Involvement of Family Members of Addicts Who Are Addicted to the Psycho Active Substance (PAS)

Due to broken family relations in the family of addicts, the non-addicted family members are very interested in the treatment of addiction. Seems to be glad to get involved through a partnership (e.g., to pick-up medication at the pharmacy, to come to see a doctor together with a patient, to control taking pills at home and to observe their behavior.

This model of treatment brings several benefits:

- Family psycho-education is included in our intervention (information about PAS and substance abuse are provided to non-addicted family members).
- The stigma is reduced or eliminated as well as the fear of this disease. Initially, it is profoundly important for establishing trust in relationship between family members and addict who begins to heal.
- No longer need to look for a daily dose of opiates and for the money that he or she must have to get it. Now, the patient stays at home, sober and of good behavior, prepared for the activities within the family that one had previously avoided.
- The treatment partner is directly controlling taking pills, which support renewal of the forgotten emotional binds between "parent and a child."

- The appetite improves and the patient gain in weight, while the whole family is having meal together their relationships improve too.
- The addict is forbidden to behave improperly, to take pills on their own, and no offence is to be made. If this happens, a partner in the therapy is obliged to report to the physician in order to detect and mediate in problem solving.
- The patient is prohibited to possess a Buprenorphine/Naloxone pill. Having Buprenorphine/Naloxone in a pocket is considered as to be possession with the intent to distribute in black market on the street. According to the agreement with a police, if this is a case, it is treated as a serious offense that must be reported and prosecuted [12].

Reliable Coordination with Pharmacy

There is a telephone connection between authorized psychiatrists who prescribe recipes with the pharmacy authorized for Buprenorphine/Naloxone procurement and its distribution.

In case of any doubts, the pharmacist makes a phone call to physician in charge of prescription to check details. If anything wrong is detected, medication distribution is stopped, while patient and treatment partner are referred back to physician in charge to correct mistake. The medication can not be distributed to anyone before a signed copy of documentation about regular introduction to treatment based on our doctrine is submitted. It provides the maximum level of distribution control from the pharmacy, preventing drug to be available on the black market.

Detection and Integrated Interdisciplinary Treatment of Infections of HIV, Hepatitis B and C

It is necessary that the experts that are responsible for the treatment of chronic hepatitis C in opiate addicts organize a multidisciplinary team, so the treatment would be coordinated by the Interferon of every I.V. addict positive to chronic hepatitis C from the discovery of the disease to its cure. That is the way to achieve double performance, with the treatment of opiate addiction, the additional infectious and highly harmful disease, is also cured [12].

Before the addict is considered for substitution treatment introduction, a candidate is obliged to do regular serological testing for HIV, HBV and HCV

[13] through a strict laboratory procedure required in our doctrine. If the person is positive to HIV, Hepatitis B and/or Hepatitis C, she or he is referred to the specialist for infectious diseases and hepatologist to perform a gene typization of virus and to begin an adequate antiviral therapy. Representatives from the Department for infectious diseases, Department for Internal diseases and Department for Psychiatry made a protocol of collaboration ensuring that these patients are treated from the infectious disease, which is result of intravenous opiates administration using non sterile needles. Since neuropsychiatrists are physicians in charge for introduction and addiction treatment, and additionally trained in psychotherapy, it is easy for them to detect psychological difficulties that arise in persons who began treatment with interferon, thereby quickly and properly react in time. It is known that intravenous opiate addicts with co-morbid Hepatitis C who undergo simultaneous treatment of both conditions are not prone to relapse [13]. In this way we discovered 50/195 opiate addicts hepatitis C positive. Although faced with danger of the final result if not treated in time, addicts when became aware that they were hepatitis C positive, they avoid further needed procedures leading to the inclusion of specific therapy with pegylated interferon. In this paper, the authors presented the procedure of multidisciplinary approach of treatment of hepatitis C positive opiate addicts despite their resistances they do not occur on the continuation of the procedure detecting HCV genotypes, and the inclusion of specific therapy for the treatment of hepatitis C in the clinics for infectious or internal diseases.

At the end, the authors present eleven clinical vignettes of successful treatment of hepatitis C in opiate addicts realized with multidisciplinary team. All of the treated individuals, after finished interferon treatment appeared hepatitis C negative [14].

Detection and Integrated Treatment of Dual Diagnosis

Introduction to substitution treatment with Buprenorphine/Naloxone helps in solving problems that resulted from opiate abuse, and then basic problems related to dual diagnosis appear. These are mainly presented with depression, sleep disorder, flash backs and night mares or psychotic equivalent or uncontrolled aggression that has been invisible while the person was taking drug regularly.

The key to effective treatment for clients with dual disorders is the seamless integration of psychiatric and substance abuse intervention in order to form a cohesive, unitary system of care [15]. Though the treatment is part of everyday clinical practice on the Department of psychiatry leaded from two psychiatrists, our approach is consisted from the elements of stage-wise case management for clients with dual diagnoses, in which services are provided in a manner consistent with addict's motivation to change his/her substance use behavior.

These services include a proper medication for depression, aggressiveness, hypnotics, psychotic symptoms and psychotherapeutic work, advocacy, clinical coordination and promoting rehabilitation and recovery. Both psychiatrists completed group analysis and EMDR psychotherapy, so they are competent to work with clients individual psychotherapy, psychotherapy with family members included in the treatment as partners when it is necessary and to work in the groups of addicts, or in mixed groups of addicts and their family members when we found it may help clients to understand the effects of substances on their lives, and to motivate them to work on these problems in a supportive, nonconfrontational group milieu to achieve abstinence. In our work with opiate addicts and their family members we help them to develop skills how to become more effective for establishing and deeping interpersonal relationships, managing negative emotions, overcoming stigma, and dealing with social situations involving substance use [15, 16].

Discovering the Trials and Prescribed Penal Measures, and Assisting in Serving a Quality Behavior in Court Action That Is Carried out in a Penal Institution

Our treatment model is also available for opiate addicts prior to and while serving a prison sentence. When treatment started for any treated opiate addict, we did not stop protocol of regular administration of Buprenorphine/Naloxone when any of them had to go to prison regardless how long the sentence will last. Collaboration is established with prison staffs that are in charge of medication, urine screening and escorting the patients to a regular medical assessment every 28th days. After checking the regularity of urine sample, we prescribe recipes for the next 28 days, and security officers go to pharmacy to take new quantity of Buprenorphine/Naloxon pills. In Penalty Institution (Prison) in Tuzla a hardened control during the taking of Buprenorphine/Naloxon pills has been established. Whilst taking the Buprenorphine/Naloxon pills (in the presence of medical worker and medical security service) the patient has to wait until the pill melts, and to open his mouth to show there is nothing inside. Also, frequently a surprise Urine opiate tests are conducted.

The Buprenorphine/Naloxon pills are held inside a safe, in a building inaccessible by convicted and imprisoned individuals. Daily, the medical staff gets the correct daily doses of pills, while the weekends the security gets the weekend doses [5]. It is important to emphasize that this treatment was from the resources of Institution of Health Insurance of Tuzla Canton.

As Institution for Health Insurance of Tuzla Canton changed Director, the new one did not support medical treatment during the aging prison sentences, he sent us a letter and requested from us to stop our activities that we began with our clients who were in prison.

Fortunately, we have got meaningful support from Global Fund (Switzerland) and United Nations Development Program (UNDP) for Bosnia-Herzegovina from the resources aimed to eliminate dangerousness of HIV and Hepatitis B and C infections. These Institutions supplied our University Clinical Center with enough quantities of Buprenorphine/Naloxon pills, so our clients continued to be regularly treated in this protocol, during staying in prison, and continue with it when they finish their obligations there, when they go out to freedom again [17].

Meanwhile, after implementation of continual treatment in prison in cooperation with jail officers (nurse and guards) they were surprised with surprising positive effects on overall outcomes of continual substitution therapy of opiate dependence with Buprenorphine/Naloxon. Also all of participants in this study were very satisfied with life quality during treatment in prison.

Also jail officers, family members of dependant person showed satisfaction with achieved efficacy of Buprenorphine/Naloxon eider during aging penalties [5].

Fighting Stigma and Successful Rehabilitation and Resocialization

From the first visit of opiate addicts and their family members to our Department with motivation and desire to begin opiate substitution treatment we started protocol to address the stigma that impacts medication-assisted treatment. We train patients and professionals for advocacy in every day meetings.

We educate Buprenorphine/Naloxone patients to dispel stigma and achieve better treatment outcomes. When they accept that they are former opiate addicts and regular citizens in near perspective it helps them to overcome ignorance and stigma. These protocols have the potential to end stigma and elevate medication-assisted treatment to its rightful place as the gold standard of treatment.

- With this treatment, our clients returned to their homes, continued life in their regular emotional and social roles, such as: being sons and daughters of their parents, spouses of their partners, parents of their children and friends.
- Those who have hepatitis C or B, are detected and involved in the treatment procedure with interferon, which prevents later complications of liver disease and premature death [12].
- They will not experience and die due to "overdose".
- They won't steal and distribute drug(s) in order to provide "a daily dose of opiates" that they need to survive somehow with no withdrawal.
- Those who are in trial or already prosecuted to serving a prison sentence, have a chance to continue the treatment in prison, which is supporting the abstinence and safety that they will not return to addiction and crime.
- If employed, they successfully return to their occupational roles. If unemployed, they are seeking for a regular job on the labor market. Three patients had entered university and study while taking Buprenorphine/Naloxone.
- Twelve of them got married after introduction substitution treatment, having their wives as partners in the treatment process. Based on our doctrine, the medication is taking daily at home in the presence of treatment partner, who is carefully monitoring his/her partner and regularity of treatment.
- Twenty one of addicts successfully completed treatment and continued normal drug-free life. We would like to point out that in current context of health care policy, we are spending a lot of money for the treatment of different chronic difficult to treat and/or incurable diseases using expensive methods and medicaments while results of these treatments in the perspective are inefficient (Diabetes mellitus, Blood hypertension, malignant processes and so on).

BENEFITS OF SUBSTITUTION MAINTEINANCE TREATMENT OF OPIOID DEPENDENCE WITH BUPRENORPHINE/NALOXONE METHOD

Since 27 July 2009 to present we have successfully introduced to treatment the 214 (two hundred fourteen) opiate addicts from several cantons of the Federation of Bosnia and Herzegovina, and several places from Republic of Srpska. Two addicts coming from Serbia (Valjevo) also begun with our treatment program, of which both are fully-charged being a foreign national.

According to our monthly report in February 2014, the 147 persons are enrolled in everyday treatment at home, one visit to our Department every 28 days in the presence of their partners.

Eight addicts of total of 214 who violated and broke the rules of treatment were temporarily excluded from the program, and after repentance and promises to adherence to treatment they were introduced again, following complete introduction procedure (laboratory and HIV and Hepatitis C and B serological testing) and after they signed new informed consent.

Out of 43 persons who are out of program now, 21 recovered addicts ceased use of the Buprenorphine/Naloxone and move into drug-free recovery and normal life [10]. Two patients from Sarajevo who were introduced to our program continued their treatment in Sarajevo. One patient continued his substitution therapy in Austria where he resides, but he was introduced to our program during holidays he spent in B&H. Another one from Brcko District ceased use of the drug due to a lack of finance, and his insurance does not cover the treatment in the Federation of B&H. One patient illegally escaped from BH when he invited to prison, and immigrated to Denmark in order to avoid serving a prison sentence. The others stopped treatment due to various forms of violation of treatment contract that they willingly signed. Some of them often committed crimes, including drug trafficking, and several of them are prisoners now.

Our work is also focused on individual psychotherapy model that will help overcoming psychological complaints and the reasons for relapse. Our goal is to support rehabilitation and re-socialization of all opiate addicts, to help them to increase the level of their social functionality and to achieve drug-free recovery.

A daily dose per patient was from 7.8 mg (April 2013) to 7.1 mg (January 2014), and the average daily dose of 7.7 mg for the last eight months. Knowing that the recommended daily dose of Buprenorphine/Naloxone may be from 4mg to 32 mg, our patients successfully maintained remission and abstinence with less than 1/4 of maximum dose (32 mg), which is considered to be an excellent result.

On the other hand, if we take into consideration:

- That each young people, while taking heroin, spent app. 25 Euros for illicit drug(s) supply; when we start to treat them, each of them have been moved from the street(s), not taking part in drug trafficking in an amount of app 750 Euros per person. When multiplied it with a number of treated addicts with buprenorphine/naloxone, this figure increases a hundred forty seven times. It means that the black market is loosing 110 250.00 Euros monthly and about 40 241 250.00 Euros annually.
- It is stated that in U.S., 1 US $ invested into heroin addiction is saving 10 US $.

Suboxone – An Effective Buprenorphine/ Naloxone Combination

Buprenorphine is a partial agonist at the mu-opioid receptor and an antagonist at the kappa-opioid receptor. Buprenorphine/Naloxone is a combination of buprenorphine to which antagonist naloxone is added to reduce the likelihood of content and abuse of intravenous administration of dissolved tablets. When taken sublingually, buprenorphine acts but Naloxone does not work and there has been a therapeutic effect achieved. But if Buprenorphine/Naloxone tablets are crushed and injected subcutaneously or intravenously, the effect of naloxone antagonist is overridden, causing withdrawal symptoms, in the addictive jargon known as "night time", so that addicts do not want to take it improperly, and the abuse is prevented.

According to benefit-cost analysis of opioid addiction treatment with buprenorphine and methadone, the annual treatment costs per addict in Croatia covered by health insurance are reduced twice if buprenorphine is used [18].

In the Italian analysis of the costs of buprenorphine vs methadone treatment of opiate addicts the results show that with the same action and even higher market price of buprenorphine, the latter represents a cheaper alternative of addiction treatment for the society due to shorter duration of treatment and especially flexible regime of administration (a patient is rarely coming to addiction center than in case of methadone treatment) [19].

Buprenorphine/Naloxone therapy resulted in a significant drop in the number of deaths associated with the use of medicine compared to methadone, and ten times lower number of deaths from opiate overdoses. Buprenorphine/Naloxone does not lead to the development of tolerance (no need for a constant increase in dose); it is far less addictive, and better tolerated than methadone known to cause serious cardiac arrhythmias, particularly in drug addicts with previous heart disease, disorder of mineral/salt metabolism or impairment of liver function. Also, the interruption of Buprenorphine/Naloxone therapy, if necessary, is much less complicated. This "smart drug" has far fewer interactions with other drugs compared to methadone.

Also, it reduces the possibility of illegal use unlike methadone. It is helping us to support the patient to become distant from addictive surroundings. Buprenorphine/Naloxone diminishes their stigmatization, it is well suited for take home medication, which significantly reduces the presence of patients/addicts in the waiting rooms of health facilities as well as the need for alternative treatment in so-called social institutions/communities. It is important to emphasize that the patients taking Buprenorphine/Naloxone at home have three times greater chance of employment than those involved in methadone programs. Students who interrupted their study due to opiate dependence, returned to university while in Buprenorphine/Naloxone treatment reporting on Buprenorphine/Naloxone to “clear their mind”. Some of those admitted to Buprenorphine/Naloxone therapy, who did not study previously, became interested in applying and successfully enrolled in university [20].

Buprenorphine/Naloxone is well suited for home use, and may be prescribed to the new patients, patients who are returning to a treatment program and those switching from other therapies. The experiences of institutions dealing with Buprenorphine/Naloxone treatment have shown that this is the safest and most cost-effective treatment option for opiate/heroin addicts. If therapy process is well implemented, a reconstruction of the brain function, the personality development and the improvement of the overall living conditions of addicts and their families is achieved in time. In comparison with methadone treatment, Buprenorphine/Naloxone has an advantage for after the maintenance program on an adequate daily dose, the overall capacity of drug addicts is increasing, and therefore he or she has a better chance for successful and complete quitting, maintaining abstinence without any medicine [21, 22]. Methadone more often induces tolerance, with an increasing dose of the drug required, leading to more severe clinical presentation. Therefore, after a few years despite the wish of an addict to detoxify, the chances for the establishment and maintenance of abstinence are lowered.

CONCLUSION

With introduction of medical model of substitution therapy for opiate addiction in 27 July 2009 at the Department for Psychiatry of the University Clinical Center Tuzla, we provide a new doctrinal approach that proved to be very effective. This model and approach ensure the maximum control of the drug, the elimination of almost all patterns of addictive behavior and partnership with non-addicted family members, reducing or eliminating stigma, making sobriety a way of life, and preventing social exclusion through rehabilitation and re-socialization. Establishing reliable coordination with pharmacy supports the maximum control of drug trafficking. Furthermore, this approach helps in detection and treatment of dual diagnosis and referral of HIV, hepatitis B and C patients. Knowing of the trials and penal measures to be taken, in collaboration with staff of correctional institutions this framework is assisting addicts in maintaining his or her new lifestyle and behavior while serving their sentences. he method also provides future admission to treatment of a greater number of opiate addicts caught in a trap of complex, multi-layer dependence and its somatic and psychosocial complications caused by long-term addictive and criminal behavior.

ACKNOWLEDGMENTS

The authors are grateful to all individuals and institutions that support and helped in developing of better and more modern mental health care in postwar Bosnia-Herzegovina. We thank to our clients: drug addicts, their parents, their spouses and their children, because they decided to break heroin addiction and bravely chose treatment instead of tragically consequences of dependency. We use this opportunity to thank Tommy Strandberg, Halid Hadžimusić, Björn

Lindquist and Ahmo Gerin from Örebro in Sweden and to Nedret Mujkanović, Elmir Čičkušić, Sabit Omić, Šehzada Salihbašić and Osman Sinanović for their support to this pioneer project from the first idea to its' realization. Great contribution to this treatment provided UNDP in Bosnia-Herzegovina with Global Fund resources. Particular thanks to Nerma Borčak for her contribution in the treatment of HCV infected opiate addicts who are in maintenance treatment with Suboxone®. We are thankful to all those who kindly helped the people of BH to alleviate the tragic consequences of the 1992-1995 war, particularly to Syed Arshad Husain and his team from Missouri University, Columbia, Missouri, USA.

REFERENCES

[1] Holma K, Koski-Jännes A, Raitasalo K, Blomquist J, Pervova I, Cunningham JA. Perceptions of addictions as Societal problems in Canada, Sweden, Finland and St. Petersburg, Russia. *Eur. Addict. Res.*, 2011; 17(2):106-112.

[2] Mehić-Basara N, Cerić I. Treatment of addicts in Bosnia and Herzegovina —constraints and opportunities. *Psychiatr. Danub.*, 2012;24 Suppl 3:S392-7. PubMed PMID: 23114823.

[3] Smyth BP, Fagan J, Kernan K. Outcome of heroin-dependent adolescents presenting for opiate substitution treatment. *J. Subst. Abuse. Treat.*, 2012; 42(1):35-44. doi: 10.1016/j.jsat.2011.07.007. Epub 2011 Sep 21. PubMed PMID: 21940134.

[4] Hasanović M. Odnos društvene zajednice prema problemima ovisnosti o Psihoaktivnim supstancama. In: Sinanović O (Ed.). Ovisnost o drogama - uzroci i posljedice, prevencija i liječenje. Multidisciplinarni pristup. Tuzla: Behram-begova Medresa u Tuzli i Medicinski fakultet Univerziteta u Tuzli. 2001: 167-185.

[5] Hasanović M, Kuldija A, Pajević I, Delić A, Sutović A, Avdibegović E, Stanišić D. Medical assisted treatment of opiate dependence with Buprenorphine/Naloxon (Buprenorphine/Naloxone) of heroin addicts in prison who are aging penalties. *Isues of Socia Science*, 2013; 1(1):21-32. DOI: http;//dx.doi.org/10.5296/iss.v1i1.4177

[6] Hasanović M. Islamski pristup u tretmanu alkoholizma, depresije, suicidalnosti i psihotraume. In: Sinanović O, Hafizović R, Pajević I (Eds). Duhovnost i mentalno zdravlje. Sarajevo: IP Svjetlost. 2002: 107-124.

[7] Hasanović M, Pajević I, Kuldija A, Delić A, Sutović A. Medical assisted treatment of opioid dependence with Buprenorphine/Naloxone method as prevention of social excluding Young people. European Psychiatry. 2011; 25 (Suppl. 1) 19th European Congress of Psychiatry. 12-15 March, 2011 - Vienna, Austria.

[8] Demetrovics Z, Farkas J, Csorba J, Németh A, Mervó B, Szemelyácz J, Fleischmann E, Kasai-Farkas A, Petke Z, Oroján T, Rózsa S, Rigó P, Funk S, Kapitány M, Kollár A, Rácz J. Early experience with Suboxone maintenance therapy in Hungary. *Neuropsychopharmacol Hung*, 2009; 11 (4):249- 57.

[9] Hasanović M, Hasanović Azra. Odnos islama prema problemima ovisnosti. In: Sinanović O (Ed.). Ovisnost *o drogama* - uzroci i posljedice, prevencija i liječenje. Multidisciplinarni pristup. Tuzla: Behram-begova Medresa u Tuzli i Medicinski Fakultet Univerziteta u Tuzli. 2001: 201-208.

[10] Hasanović M, Pajević I, Kuldija A, Delić A. Sutović A. Quality of life of heroin addicts and their family members improved during medical assisted treatment of opiate dependence with Buprenorphine/Naloxone (Buprenorphine/Naloxone). *British Journal of Medical and Health Sciences*, 2012; 1(1):55 -62. (October 2012).

[11] Maremmani I, Gerra G. Buprenorphine-based regimens and methadone for the Medical management of opioid dependence: selecting the appropriate drug for treatment. *Am. J. Addict.*, 2010; 19(6):557-68.

[12] Hasanović M, Pajević I, Kuldija A, Delić A, Sutović A, Avdibegović E, Aljukić N. Problems in inducing Interferon therapy of opiate addicts with Hepatitis C who are in substitution maintainance therapy with Buprenorphine/ Naloxone (Suboxone®). *International Journal of Science,* 2013; 2(10): 40-4. http://www.ijsciences.com/pub/article/310.

[13] Hasanović M, Pajević I, Kuldija A, Delić A, Sutović A. Some Epidemiological Characteristics of Opiate Addicts with Hepatitis C who are in Substitution Maintainance Therapy with Buprenorphine/Naloxone (Suboxone) in Bosnia -Herzegovina. *European Psychiatry*, The Journal of the association of European psychiatrists: 20th European Congress of Psychiatry. Abstracts on CD-ROM, 2012; 27(Suppl. 1): P-35. 3-6 March - Prague-Czech Republic. http://www.europsy-journal.com/article /S0924-9338%2812%2974202-5/abstract.

[14] Hasanović M, Pajević I, Kuldija A, Delić A, Sutović A, Avdibegović E, Aljukić N, Šabić Dž. Successful treatment with Interferon therapy of Hepatitis C positive opiate addicts who are in substitution maintenance

therapy with Buprenorphine/Naloxone (Suboxone®). European Psychiatry, The Journal of the association of European psychiatrists: 22st European Congress of Psychiatry. Abstracts on the USB key. 2014; 29(Suppl. 1). EPA-0908. 1-4 March 2014 Munich - Germany.

[15] Mueser TK, Noordsy LD, Drake ER, Fox L. Integrated Treatment for dual disorders - A guide to effective practice. New York: The Guildford Press. 2003.

[16] Hasanović M, Šabić Dž, Kuldija A, Pajević I. Integrative complex personalized treatment of dual diagnoses of opiate drug addict person who is treated with maintenance substitution opiate therapy with buprenorphine/naloxone (Buprenorphine/Naloxone)-Case report. European Psychiatry, *The Journal of the association of European psychiatrists:* 22st European Congress of Psychiatry. Abstracts on the USB key. 2014; 29(Suppl. 1). EPA-0904. 1-4 March 2014 Munich - Germany.

[17] Šeremet N, Drinić A, Babić Dž. UNDP's support to OST program for addicts through the grant funded by the Global Fund. Book of Abstracts of 3rd Congress of psychiatrists of Bosnia-Herzegovina with international participation. Tuzla, 12th -14th October 2012. Tuzla, Psychiatric Association of Bosnia-Herzegovina. p:165.

[18] Čulig J & Sakoman S. Farmakoekonomska analiza ukupnih troškova liječenja ovisnika o opijatima u kojih se liječenje ovisnosti provodi buprenorfinom, odnosno metadonom. Zavod za javno zdravstvo grada Zagreba. 2005.

[19] Colombo LG, Faillace G, Ferdico M. Analiza troškova (cijene) buprenorfina u odnosu na metadon (buprenorfin vs. metadon) u liječenju ovisnika o opijatima. *Farmaeconomia e percorsi terapeutici,* 2003; 4 (4): 185-192.

[20] Ling W, Jacobs P, Hillhouse M, Hasson A, Thomas C, Freese T, Sparenborg S, McCarty D, Weiss R, Saxon A, Cohen A, Straus M, Brigham G, Liu D, McLaughlin P, Tai B. From research to the real world: buprenorphine in the decade of the Clinical Trials Network. J. Subst. Abuse, Treat. 2010; 38 (Suppl. 1):S53-60.

[21] Kakko J, Svanborg KD, Kreek MJ, Heilig M. 1-year retention and social function after buprenorphine-assisted relapse prevention treatment for heroin dependence in Sweden: a randomised, placebo-controlled trial. Lancet. 2003 Feb22;361(9358): 662 -8. PubMed PMID: 12606177.

[22] Kakko J, Grönbladh L, Svanborg KD, von Wachenfeldt J, Rück C, Rawlings B, Nilsson LH, Heilig M. A stepped care strategy using buprenorphine and methadone versus conventional methadone maintenance in heroin dependence: a randomized controlled trial. *Am. J. Psychiatry,* 2007;164(5):797-803. PubMed PMID: 17475739.

Index

A

B

C

D

E

F

G

H

I

J

K

L

M

N

O

P

Q

R

S

T

U